VOL 1

PATIENT CARE TECHNICIAN

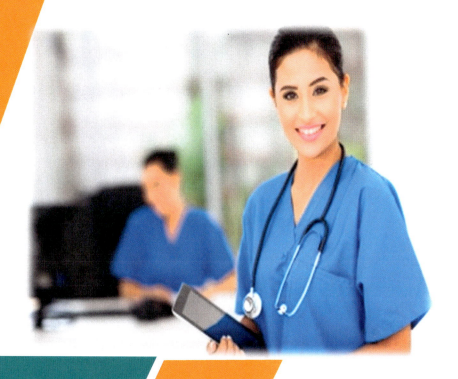

Exam Study Guide

Jane John-Nwankwo RN, MSN

PATIENT CARE TECHNICIAN EXAM STUDY GUIDE:

Volume One

Copyright © 2017 by Jane John-Nwankwo RN, MSN

All rights reserved. No part of this book may be reproduced or transmitted in any form or by any means without written permission from the author.

ISBN-13: 978-1545067284

ISBN-10: 1545067287

Printed in the United States of America.

DEDICATION

To my loving husband, John U Nwankwo Ph.D.

OTHER TITLES FROM THE SAME AUTHOR:

01 Medication Technician Study guide

02 Nurses' Romance Series

03 CNA Exam Prep: Nurse Assistant Practice Test Questions. Vol. 1 & 2

04 Home Health Aide Training Manual

05 IV Therapy & Blood Withdrawal Review Questions

06 Medical Assistant Test Preparation

07 EKG Test Prep

08 Phlebotomy Test Prep Vol 1, 2, & 3

09 The Home Health Aide Textbook

10 How to make a million in nursing

And Many More Books

Visit www.healthcarepracticetest.com

www.janejohn-nwankwo.com

Simply Search Jane John-Nwankwo on Amazon

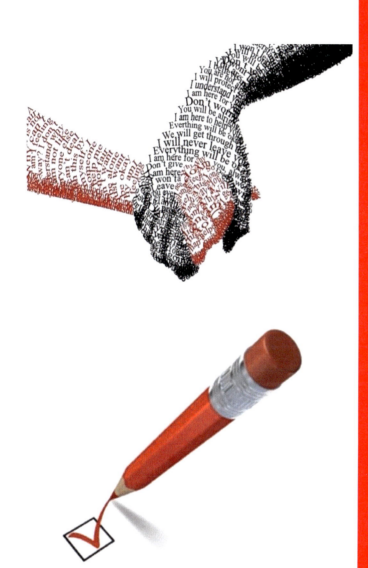

Contents

SECTION 01
PATIENT CARE TECHNICIAN DUTIES

SECTION 02
EKG REVIEW

Section One

General Information For The Patient Care Technician

Patient Care Technicians, also known as nursing assistants, geriatric aides, unlicensed assistive personnel, or hospital attendants, perform routine tasks under the supervision of nursing and medical staff.

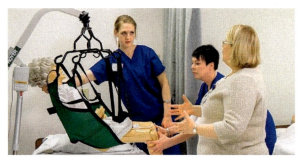

They answer patients' call lights, deliver messages, serve meals, make beds, and help patients eat, dress, and bathe. PCTs also may provide skin care to patients; take their temperatures, pulse rate, respiration rate, and blood pressure; and help patients get in and out of bed and walk. They also may escort patients to operating and examining rooms, keep patients' rooms neat, set up equipment, store and move supplies, or assist with some procedures. They observe patients' physical, mental, and emotional conditions and report any change to the nursing or medical staff.

PCTs help care for physically or mentally ill, injured, disabled, or infirm individuals confined to hospitals, nursing care facilities, and mental health settings. Home health aides' duties are similar, but they work in patients' homes or residential care facilities. The main difference between patient care technicians and nurse Assistants is the inclusion of phlebotomy and EKG technician duties in their roles. Hence a patient care technician can work under nurses or as a medical assistant, under doctors.

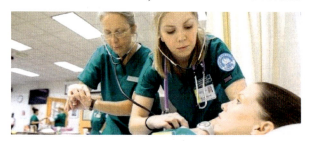

PCTs can work as nurse assistants, phlebotomists, EKG Technicians, etc.

Some states would allow patient care technicians to work as home health aides while some states like California would require a specific certification as a home health aide. Check your state policies.

Working Conditions

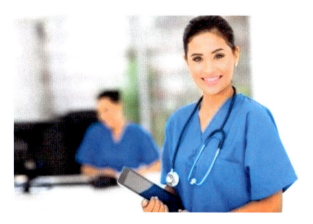

Most full-time patient care technicians work about 40 hours a week. However, since some patients need care 24 hours a day, some PCTs work evenings, nights, weekends, and holidays. Many work part time. PCTs spend many hours standing and walking, and they often face heavy workloads. Because they may have to move patients in and out of bed or help them stand or walk, aides must guard against back injury. PCTs also may face hazards from minor infections and major diseases, such as hepatitis, but can avoid infections by following proper procedures.

PCTs often have unpleasant duties, such as emptying bedpans and changing soiled bed linens. The patients they care for may be disoriented, irritable, or uncooperative.

Employment

Some employers provide classroom instruction for newly hired PCTs, while others rely exclusively on informal on-the-job instruction from a licensed nurse or an experienced tech. Such training may last several days to a few months. From time to time, PCTs also may attend lectures, workshops, and in-service training.

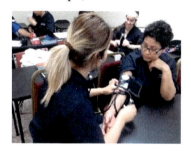

These occupations can offer individuals an entry into the world of work. The flexibility of night and weekend hours also provides high school and college students a chance to work during the school year.

Applicants should be tactful, patient, understanding, emotionally stable, and dependable and should have a desire to help people. They also should be able to work as part of a team, have good communication skills, and be willing to perform repetitive, routine tasks.

PCTs must be in good health. A physical examination, including State-regulated tests such as those for tuberculosis, may be required.

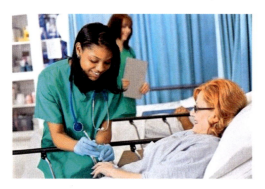

JOB OUTLOOK

Numerous job openings for patient care technicians will arise from a combination of fast employment growth and high replacement needs. High replacement needs in this large occupation reflect modest entry requirements, low pay, high physical and emotional demands, and lack of opportunities for advancement. For these same reasons, many people are unwilling to perform the kind of work required by the occupation. Therefore, persons who are interested in, and suited for, this work should have excellent job opportunities.

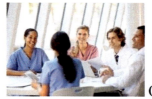

Overall employment of patient care technicians is projected to grow for all occupations through the year 2020, although individual occupational growth rates will vary. Employment of PCTs is expected to grow the fastest, as a result of both growing demand for home healthcare services from an aging population and efforts to contain healthcare costs by moving patients out of hospitals and nursing care facilities as quickly as possible. Consumer preference for care in the home and improvements in medical technologies for in-home treatment also will contribute to faster-than-average employment growth for PCTs.

The PCT Working in a Doctor's Office

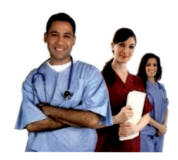

Patient Care Technicians perform routine tasks in a wide variety of locations such as hospitals, medical offices, and clinics. The PCT should only perform the range of activities that is within their scope of practice. They should not be confused with physician assistants, who examine, diagnose, and treat patients under the direct supervision of a physician. Clinical duties vary according to State law and include taking medical histories and recording vital signs, explaining treatment procedures to patients, preparing patients for examination, and assisting the physician during the examination.

PCTs working in a doctor's office collect and prepare laboratory specimens or perform basic laboratory tests on the premises, dispose of contaminated supplies, and sterilize medical instruments. They instruct patients about medications and special diets, prepare and administer medications as directed by a physician, authorize drug refills as directed, telephone prescriptions to a pharmacy, draw blood, prepare patients for x rays, take electrocardiograms, remove sutures, and change dressings.

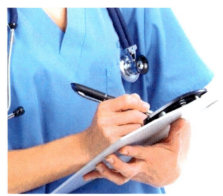

THE MEDICAL HISTORY

Parts of the patient's medical history are:

- *Chief Complaint (CC):* The reason why the patient came to see the physician.

- *History of Present Illness (HPI):* This is an explanation of the chief complaint to determine the onset of the illness; associated symptoms; what the patient has done to treat the condition, etc. Past, Family and Social History (PFSH):

- *Past Medical History*: includes all health problems, major illnesses, surgeries the patient has had, current medications complete with reasons for taking them, and allergies.

- *Family History:* summary of health problems of siblings, parents, and other blood relatives that could alert the physician to hereditary and/or familial diseases.

- *Social History:* includes marital status, occupation, educational attainment, hobbies, use of alcohol, tobacco, drugs, and lifestyles.

Review of Systems - this is an orderly and systematic check of each organ and system of the body by questions. Both positive and pertinent negative findings are documented. The ROS, in conjunction with the physical examination, helps elicit information that is essential to the diagnosis of patient's condition.

VITAL SIGNS

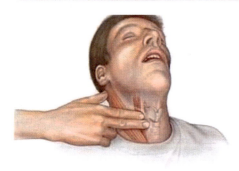

Reflect the functions of three body processes necessary for life:

- Body temperature
- Respiration
- Heart function

The four vital signs of body function are:

 Temperature

 Pulse

 Respiration

 Blood pressure

TEMPERATURE

Body temperature is a balance between heat production and heat loss in conjunction with each other, maintained and regulated by the hypothalamus.

Thermometers are used to measure temperature using the Fahrenheit and Centigrade or Celsius scale. Temperature sites are the following: mouth, rectum, ear (tympanic membrane), and the axilla (underarm). The normal ranges for each site are:

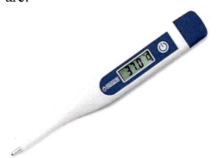

Site **Normal Range**

Rectal 98.6F to 100.6F (37.0C to 38.1C)

Oral 97.6F to 99.6F (36.5C to 37.5C)

Axillary 96.6F to 98.6F (35.9C to 37.0C)

Tympanic Membrane 98.6F (37C)

Some terms used to describe body temperature are:

❖ **Febrile** – presence of fever

❖ **Afebrile** – absence of fever

Fever – elevated body temperature beyond normal range. Types of fever are:

Intermittent: fluctuating fever that returns to or below baseline then rises again.

Remittent: fluctuating fever that remains elevated; it does not return to baseline temperature.

Continuous: a fever that remains constant above the baseline; it does not fluctuate.

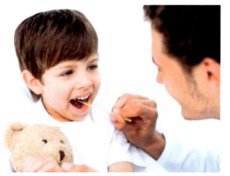

Oral temperature is the most common method of measurement; however, it is not taken from the following patients:

- infants and children less than six years old
- patients who has had surgery or facial, neck, nose, or mouth injury
- those receiving oxygen
- those with nasogastric tubes
- patients with convulsive seizure
- hemiplegic patients
- patients with altered mental status

Wait for 30 minutes to take the oral temperature in patients who have just finished eating, drinking, or smoking. When taking the temperature, leave the thermometer in the patient's mouth for 3-5 minutes or as required by agency policy.

Rectal temperature is taken when oral temperature is not feasible. However, it is not taken from the following patients:

❖ patients with heart disease

❖ patients with rectal disease or disorder or has had rectal surgery

❖ patients with diarrhea

It is taken with the patient in a side-lying position and the thermometer and the patient's hip is held throughout the procedure so the thermometer is not lost in the rectum or broken.

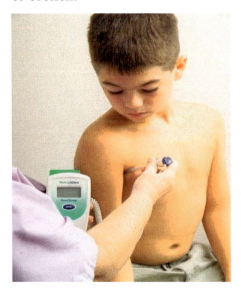

Axillary temperature is the least accurate and is taken only when no other temperature site can be used. The axilla, (the underarm) should be clean and dry and the thermometer should be held in place for 5-10 minutes or as required by the facility policy.

Tympanic temperature is useful for children and confused patients because of the speed of operation of the tympanic thermometer. A covered probe is gently inserted into the ear canal and temperature is measured within seconds (1–3 seconds). It is not used if the patient has an ear disorder or ear drainage.

PULSE

The normal adult pulse rate ranges between 60 and 100 beats per minute. The site most commonly used for taking pulse is the radial artery found in the wrist on the same side as the thumb. It is felt with the first two or three fingers (never with the thumb) and usually taken for 30 seconds multiplied by two to get the rate per minute. If the rate is unusually fast or slow, however, count it for 60 seconds.

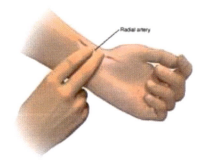

The apical pulse is a more accurate measurement of the heart rate and it is taken over the apex of the heart by auscultation using the stethoscope. It is used for patients with irregular heart rate and for infants and small children.

RESPIRATION

When measuring respiration, respiratory characteristics such as rate, rhythm, and depth are taken into account. Rate is the number of respirations per minute. The normal range for adults is 12 to 20 per minute. One inspiration (inhale) and one expiration (exhale) counts as one respiration. It is counted for 30 seconds multiplied by two or for a full minute.

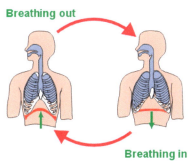

Some rate abnormalities are the following:

Apnea – this is a temporary complete absence of breathing which may be a result of a reduction in the stimuli to the respiratory centers of the brain.

Tachypnea – this is a respiration rate of greater than 40/min. It is transient in the newborn and maybe caused by the hysteria in the adult.

Bradypnea – decrease in numbers of respirations. This occurs during sleep. It may also be due to certain diseases.

Respiratory rhythm refers to the pattern of breathing. It can vary with age: infants have an irregular rhythm while adults have regular.

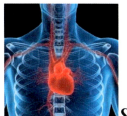

Some abnormalities in the rhythm are the following:

Cheyne-Stokes – this is a regular pattern of irregular breathing rate.

Orthopnea – this is difficulty or inability to breath unless in an upright position.

Depth of respiration refers to the amount of air that is inspired and expired during each respiration. Some abnormalities in the depth of respirations are the following:

Hypoventilation: state in which reduced amount of air enters the lungs resulting in decreased oxygen level and increased carbon dioxide level in blood. It can be due to breathing that is too shallow, or too slow, or to diminished lung function.

Hyperpnea: abnormal increase in the depth and rate of breathing.

Hyperventilation: state in which there is an increased amount of air entering the lungs.

BLOOD PRESSURE

This is the measurement of the amount of force exerted by the blood on the peripheral arterial walls and is expressed in millimeters (mm) of mercury (Hg). The measurement consist of two components: the highest (systole) and lowest (diastole) amount of pressure exerted during the cardiac cycle.

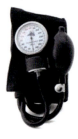

A stethoscope and sphygmomanometer of either aneroid or mercury type are used. The size of the cuff of the sphygmomanometer will depend on the circumference of the limb and not the age of the patient. The width of the inflatable bag within the cuff should be about 40% of this circumference – 12 cm to 14 cm in an average adult. The length of the bag should be about 80% of this circumference – almost long enough to encircle the arm. Cuffs that are too short or narrow may give falsely high readings, e.g. a regular cuff on an obese arm may lead to a false diagnosis of hypertension.

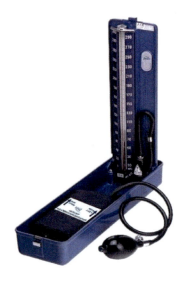

The inflatable bag is centered over the brachial artery with the lower border about 2.5cm above the antecubital crease. The cuff is positioned at heart level. If the brachial artery is far below the heart level the blood pressure will appear falsely high. If the brachial artery is far above heart level, blood pressure will appear falsely low.

Blood pressure is taken by determining first the palpatory systolic pressure over the brachial artery. Then with the bell of the stethoscope over the brachial artery, the cuff is inflated again to about 30 mm Hg above the palpatory systolic pressure and deflated slowly, allowing the pressure to drop at a rate of about 2 to 3 mmHg per second. Note the level at which you hear the sounds of at least two consecutive beats. This is the systolic pressure. Continue to lower the pressure slowly until the sounds become muffled and then disappear. Then deflate the cuff rapidly to zero. The disappearance point, which is usually only a few mmHg below the muffling point, marks the generally accepted diastolic pressure. Both the systolic and diastolic pressure levels are read the nearest 2 mmHg.

Common errors in blood pressure measurements:

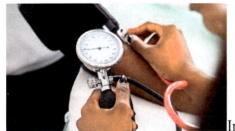

Improper cuff size. Cuffs that are too short or narrow may give falsely high readings. Using a regular cuff on an obese arm may lead to a false diagnosis of hypertension. For an obese arm, select a cuff with a larger than standard bag.

The arm is not at heart level. If the brachial artery is much below the heart level, the blood pressure will appear falsely high. Conversely, if the artery is much above heart level, blood pressure will appear falsely low. A 13.6 cm difference between arterial and cardiac levels produces a blood pressure error of 10mmHg.

Cuff is not completely deflated before use. Deflation of the cuff is faster than 2-3 mmHg per second. Rapid deflation will lead to underestimation of the systolic and overestimation of the diastolic pressure.

The cuff is re-inflated during the procedure without allowing the arm to rest for 1-2 minute between readings. Repetitive inflation of the cuff can result in venous congestion, which could make the sound less audible producing artifactually low systolic and high diastolic pressure.

Improper Cuff Placement.

Defective equipment. A bag that balloons outside the cuff leads to falsely high readings.

Anthropometric Measurements

The term anthropometric refers to comparative measurements of the body. They are used as indicators of the state of health and well-being of the patient and are often included in the initial measurement of vital signs. Anthropometric measurements require precise measuring techniques to be valid.

Length, height, weight, weight-for-length, and head circumference (length is used in infants and toddlers, rather than height, because they are unable to stand) are used to assess growth and development in infants, children and adolescents. Individual measurements are usually compared to reference standards on a growth chart.

The Physical Examination

The four principles of physical examination are:

Inspection: which provides an enormous amount of information. The observer uses observation to detect significant physical features or objective data. This method focuses on certain aspects of the patient:

- General appearance
- State of nutrition
- Body habitus
- Symmetry
- Posture and gait
- Speech

Palpation: The examiner uses the sense of touch to determine the characteristics of an organ system.

Percussion - This involves tapping or striking the body, usually with the fingers or a small hammer to determine the position, size and density of the underlying organ or tissue.

Auscultation - This involves listening to sounds produced by internal organs. It is usually done to evaluate the heart, lungs, and the abdomen.

The Patient Care Technician's role in the physical examination:

1. Room preparation
2. Patient preparation
3. Assisting the physician

To make a diagnosis, the physician utilizes three sources: the patient's health history, the physical examination, and laboratory tests. The role of the Certified PCT during a physical examination greatly depends upon the discretion of the physician. Commonly, the Patient Care Technician will prepare the patient which consists of explanation and preparation, positioning, draping, vital signs, venipuncture and EKG. The PCT may also prepare the room by assembling the needed instrument and equipment for the physical examination.

Positioning a Patient for Examination or Treatment

When performing an examination, treatment, tests or to obtain specimens, patients are put in special positions.

The Horizontal Recumbent Position is used for most physical examinations. The patient lies on his/her back with legs extended. Arms may be above the head, alongside the body or folded on the chest.

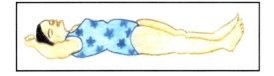

Figure 1-1. Horizontal recumbent position.

The Dorsal Recumbent Position is when the patient is on his/her back with knees flexed and soles of the feet flat on the bed. The PCT will need to fold a sheet once across the chest and fold a second sheet crosswise over the thighs and legs so that genital area is easily exposed.

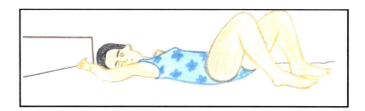

Figure 1-2. Dorsal recumbent position

The Fowler's Position is used to promote drainage or to ease breathing. A sitting or semi-sitting position where the back of the examination table is elevated to either 45 degrees (Semi-Fowler's) or 90 degrees (High- Fowler's). The knees maybe raised slightly by placing a pillow underneath, but usually the legs rest flat on the table. . The patient may need a foot support. This position is usually used for patients with cardiovascular or respiratory problems, and for the examination of the upper body and head.

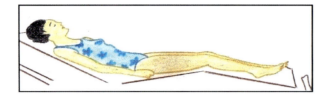

Figure 1-3. Fowler's Position.

The Dorsal Lithotomy Position is used for examination of pelvic organs. This position is similar to the dorsal recumbent position, except that the patient's legs are well separated and thighs are acutely flexed. The feet are usually placed in stirrups and a folded sheet or bath blanket is placed crosswise over thighs and legs so that genital area is easily exposed. Keep the patient covered as much as possible.

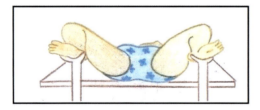

The Prone Position is used to examine the spine and back. The patient lies on his/her abdomen with head turned to one side for comfort, the arms may be above head or alongside the body. Cover with sheet or bath blanket. This position is used in the examination of the posterior aspect of the body, including the back or spine. NOTE: An unconscious patient or one with an abdominal incision or breathing difficulty usually cannot lie in this position.

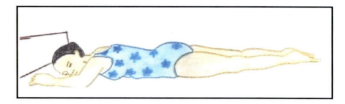

Figure 1-5. Prone position.

The Sim's Position is used for rectal examination. The patient is on his/her left side with the right knee flexed against the abdomen and the left knee slightly flexed. The left arm is behind the body; the right arm is placed comfortably. NOTE: Patient with leg injuries or arthritis usually cannot assume this position.

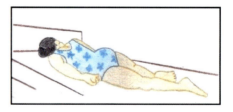

Figure 1-6. Sim's position.

The Knee-Chest Position is used for rectal and vaginal examinations and as treatment to bring the uterus into normal position. The patient is on his/her knees with his/her chest resting on the bed and elbows resting on the bed or arms above head. The head is turned to one side. The thighs are straight and lower legs are flat on the bed. NOTE: Do not leave patient alone; he/she may become dizzy, faint, and fall.

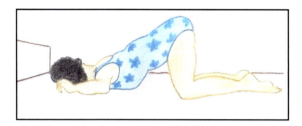

Figure 1-7. Knee-chest position.

Trendelenburg position – The patient is placed flat on the back, face up, the knees flexed and legs hanging off the end of the table, with the legs and feet supported by a footboard. The table is positioned with the head 45 degrees lower than the body. This position is used primarily for surgical procedures of pelvis and abdomen.

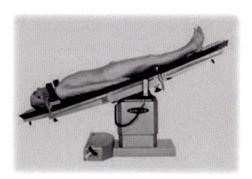

SAFETY

Safety hazards abound in the healthcare setting, many of which can cause serious injury or disease. The Occupational Safety and Health Administration (OSHA) is responsible for the identification of the various hazards present in the workplace and for the creation of rules and regulations to minimize exposure to such hazards. Employers are mandated to institute measures that will assure safe working conditions and health workers have the obligation to know and follow those measures.

Safety rules are usually based on common sense. Most accidents occur when these rules are neglected, overlooked or ignored.

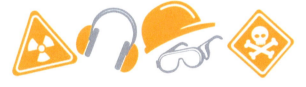

Accidents generally occur when safety is compromised because of haste and secondary shortcuts. These shortcuts can lead to personal injury and equipment damage. When an accident occurs, it must be reported to your supervisor immediately. Trying to cover up the incident can lead to serious, even disastrous results.

HAZARDS

A. Physical Hazards

- Electrical Safety Regulations
- Use only ground plugs that have been approved by Underwriters' Laboratory
- (UL).
- Never use extension cords.
- Avoid electrical circuit overloading.
- Inspect all cords and plugs periodically for damage.
- Use a surge protector on all sensitive electronic devices.
- Before servicing, UNPLUG the device from the electrical outlet.
- Use signs and/or labels to indicate high voltage or electrical hazards.

B. Chemical Hazards

- Chemical Safety Regulations
- If the skin or eyes come in contact with any chemicals, immediately wash the area
- with water for at least 5 minutes.
- Store flammable or volatile chemicals in a well-ventilated area.
- After use, immediately recap all bottles containing toxic substances.
- Label all chemicals with the required Material Safety Data Sheet (MDSD)
- information.

C. Biological Hazards

Biological Safety Regulations

1. Disinfect the laboratory work area before and after each use when dealing with biologicals.
2. Never draw a specimen through a pipette by mouth. This technique is not permitted in the laboratory.
3. Always wear gloves.
4. Sterilize specimens and any other contaminated materials and/or dispose of them through incineration.
5. Wash hands thoroughly before and after every procedure.

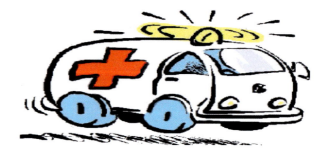

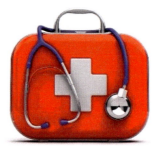

The ability to recognize and react quickly to an emergency

may be the difference of life or death for the patient. As patients react differently to various situations, it is important for all healthcare professionals to be prepared in an emergency.

External Hemorrhage: controlling the bleeding is most effectively accomplished by elevating the affected part above heart level and applying direct pressure to the wound. Do not attempt to elevate a broken extremity as this could cause further damage.

Shock occurs when there is insufficient return of blood flow to the heart, resulting in inadequate supply of oxygen to all organs and tissues of the body.' Patients experiencing trauma may go into shock and for some patients, seeing their own blood may induce shock.

Common Symptoms:

- Pale, cold, clammy skin
- Rapid, weak pulse
    - Increased, shallow breathing rate
    - Expressionless face/staring eyes.

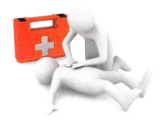

First Aid for Shock:

- Maintain an open airway for the victim
- Call for assistance
- Keep the victim lying down with the head lower than the rest of the body
- Attempt to control bleeding or cause of shock (if known)
- Keep the victim warm until help arrives

Cardiopulmonary Resuscitation. Most healthcare institutions require their professionals to be certified in CPR. It is important for all professionals to maintain all certifications acquired.

Infection Control/Chain of Infection

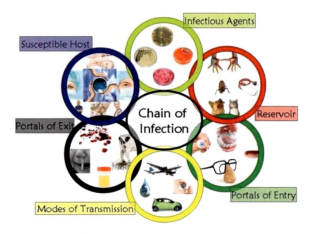

This consists of links, each of which is necessary for the infectious disease to spread. Infection control is based on the fact that the transmission of infectious diseases will be prevented or stopped when any level in the chain is broken or interrupted.

Agent --------------- Mode of transmission ------------ Susceptible host portal of exit portal of entry

Agents– are infectious microorganisms that can be classified into groups namely: viruses, bacteria, fungi, and parasites. When infectious diseases are identified according to the specific disease-causing microorganism, the disease may be prevented with the use of anti-infective drugs or infection control practices.

Portal of exit –the method by which an infectious agent leaves its reservoir.

Standard Precautions and Transmission-Based Precautions are control measures aimed at preventing the spread of the disease as infectious agents exit the reservoir.

Mode of transmission –specific ways in which microorganisms travel from the reservoir to the susceptible host. There are five main types of mode of transmission:

❖ Contact: direct and indirect
❖ Droplet
❖ Airborne
❖ Common vehicle
❖ Vectorborne

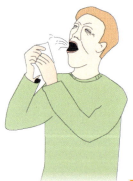

Portal of Entry

Allows the infectious agent access to the susceptible host. Common entry sites are broken skin, mucous membranes, and body systems exposed to the external environment such as the respiratory, gastrointestinal, and reproductive. Methods such as sterile wound care, transmission-based precautions, and aseptic technique limit the transmission of the infectious agents.

Susceptible host – The infectious agent enters a person who is not resistant or immune. Control at this level is directed towards the identification of the patients at risk, treat their underlying condition for susceptibility, or isolate them from the reservoir.

Medical Asepsis

Best defined as ―the destruction of pathogenic microorganisms after they leave the body.‖ It also involves environmental hygiene measures such as equipment cleaning and disinfection procedures. Methods of medical asepsis are Standard Precautions and

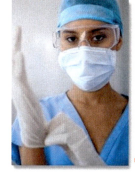

Transmission-Based Precautions

Disinfection. This procedure used in medical asepsis using various chemicals that can be used to destroy many pathogenic microorganisms. Since chemicals can irritate skin and mucous membranes, they are used only on inanimate objects.

The least expensive and most readily available disinfectant for surfaces such as countertops is a 1:10 solution of household bleach. Boiling water (temperature of 212 F) is considered a form of disinfection, but use of it in today‘s medical setting is limited to items that:

1. will not be used in invasive procedures;
2. will not be inserted into body orifices nor be used in a sterile procedure.

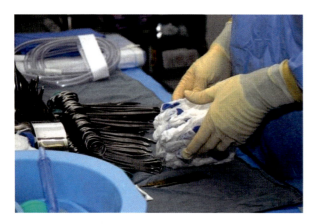

Surgical Asepsis

All microbial life, pathogens and nonpathogens, are destroyed before an invasive procedure is performed. Surgical asepsis and sterile technique are often used interchangeably.

Four Methods of Sterilization

1. Gas sterilization: often used for wheelchairs and hospital beds. Useful in hospitals, but costly for the office.

2. Dry heat sterilization: requires higher temperature that steam sterilization but longer exposure times. Used for instruments that easily corrodes.

3. Chemical sterilization - uses the same chemical used for chemical disinfection, but the exposure time is longer.

4. Steam sterilization (autoclave) - uses steam under pressure to obtain high temperature of 250-254F with exposure times of 20-40 minutes depending on the item being sterilized.

HANDWASHING

Hand washing is the most important means of preventing the spread of infection. A routine hand wash procedure uses plain soap to remove soil and transient bacteria. Hand antisepsis requires the use of antimicrobial soap to remove, kill or inhibit transient microorganisms. It is important that all healthcare personnel learn proper hand washing procedures.

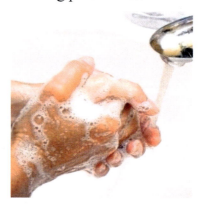

BARRIER PROTECTION

Protective clothing provides a barrier against infection. Used properly, it will provide protection to the person wearing it; disposed of properly it will assist in the spread of infection. Learning how to put on and remove protective clothing is vital to insure the health and wellness of the person wearing the PPE. PPE's or personal protective equipment includes:

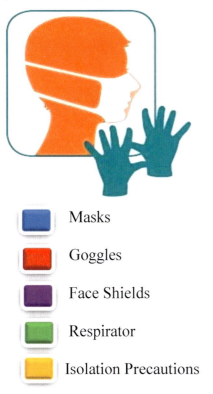

- Masks
- Goggles
- Face Shields
- Respirator
- Isolation Precautions

For many years, the CDC recommended universal precautions, which is a method of infection control that assumed that all human blood and body fluids were potentially infectious. The CDC issued a revised guideline consisting of two tiers or levels of precautions: Standard Precautions and Transmission-Based Precautions.

STANDARD PRECAUTIONS

This is an infection control method designed to prevent direct contact with blood and other body fluids and tissues by using barrier protection and work control practices. Under the standard precautions, all patients are presumed to be infective for blood-borne pathogens. Infection control practices to be used with all patients. These replace universal precautions and body substance isolation. They are used when there is a possibility of contact with any of the following:

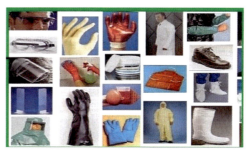

✓ Blood

- ✓ All body fluids, secretions, and excretions (except sweat), regardless of whether or not they contain visible blood
- ✓ Nonintact skin
- ✓ Mucous membranes designed to reduce the risk of transmission of microorganisms from both
- ✓ Recognized and unrecognized sources of infections.

The standard precautions are:

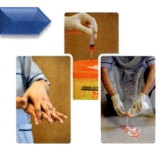

Wear gloves when collecting and handling blood, body fluids, or tissue specimen. Wear face shields when there is a danger for splashing on mucous membranes. Dispose of all needles and sharp objects in puncture-proof containers without recapping.

Transmission- Based Precautions the second tier of precautions and are to be used when the patient is known or suspected of being infected with contagious disease. They are to be used in addition to standard precautions.

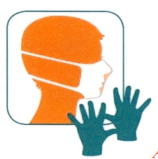

All types of isolation are condensed into three categories:

Contact Precautions: Are designed to reduce the risk of transmission of microorganisms by direct or indirect contact. Direct-contact transmission involves skin-to-skin contact and physical transfer of microorganisms to a susceptible host from an infected or colonized person. Indirect-contact transmission involves contact with a contaminated intermediate object in the patient's environment.

Airborne Precautions: are designed to reduce the risk of airborne transmission of infectious agents. Microorganisms carried in this manner can be dispersed widely by air currents and may become inhaled by or deposited on a susceptible host within the same room or over a longer distance from the source patient. Special air handling and ventilation are required to prevent airborne transmission.

Contact Precautions: are designed to reduce the risk of transmission of microorganisms by direct or indirect contact. Direct-contact transmission involves skin-to-skin contact and physical transfer of microorganisms to a susceptible host from an infected or colonized person. Indirect-contact transmission involves contact with a contaminated intermediate object in the patient's environment.

Airborne Precautions: are designed to reduce the risk of airborne transmission of infectious agents. Microorganisms carried in this manner can be dispersed widely by air currents and may become inhaled by or deposited on a susceptible host within the same room or over a longer distance from the source patient. Special air handling and ventilation are required to prevent airborne transmission.

Errors in Medication

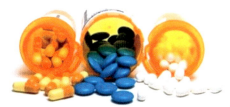

There has been a tremendous amount of research on medication errors, beginning with a study that established the fact that medication errors are a much bigger problem than was actually realized (Flynn, n.d.). Errors in medication administration were employed by researchers to study the output quality of drug distribution systems in the 1960s at the time of development of the unit dose drug distribution system.

These errors were considered an important indicator of drug therapy quality for the patient. Research on devices that perform automatic drug dispensing has shown that errors are still a common occurrence (Flynn, n.d.). Errors of medication history, such as the omission of drugs, are common.

These errors can bring harm to the patient. Moreover, hypersensitivity reactions are not explored in detail or are improperly documented, which may help in a drug being avoided unnecessarily. In addition, clinical specialty, specific drugs and polypharmacy can influence the risks of errors in medication history. Some of the reasons for the common occurrence of medication errors upon admission to hospitals include the inability of patients to accurately report their drug history. They also do not bring their previous medications or a list of those medications along with them (FitzGerald, 2009).

Principles of Medication Administration

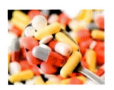

Regardless of the type of medication, certain basic principles dictate the process of medication administration. As part of these principles, PCTs are required to talk to their patients and communicate what will be done before the medication is administered. Any question that the patient may have should be clearly addressed by the professional or directed to the licensed nurse or physician overshadowing them.

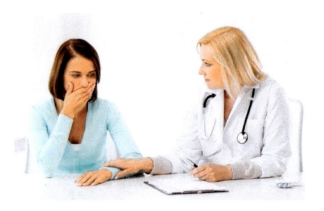

They need to help the patients in getting involved in the process of medication administration. They also need to provide privacy to the patients. The process of medication administration should be given complete and undivided attention and should be carried out in an area that is free from distraction. PCTs need to maintain cleanliness and hygiene, and should wash their hands prior to and after the administration of medication. Clayton (2012) elaborated the principles of medication administration and safety as follows:

Standards of Care, Basic Requirements and Patient Charts

The standards of care are developed by state as well as federal law in addition to the Joint Commission and professional organizations involved in patient care and treatment. PCTs are required to be familiar with the contents of the nurse practice act and any legislation that dictates their profession. The law of each state has certain limitations regarding the administration of medication. Separate policies are also provided by the healthcare institutions. Knowing and following these are the duties of PCTs and all other professionals.

While administering a medication, a PCT should have the certification and permission to practice, and a policy statement authorizing the act. He should understand the patient's symptoms and diagnosis that correlate with the rationale of the administration of the medication.

He should know why the particular drug administration has been ordered, its expected outcome, dilution, dosing, rate of administration, route of administration, expected adverse effects and contraindications. He should also be able to calculate, prepare and administer the drug accurately, apart from assessing the patient to detect any therapeutic or adverse effect the medication may have induced. The professional administering the medication should actively participate in educating the family of the patient and the patient himself regarding the treatment and discharge of the patient. In many states, this is the duty of the registered or Licensed Vocational Nurse.

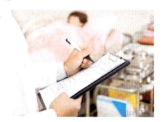

Patient charts are records that provide information to all the healthcare team members about the status of the patient, his progress and care. These are legal documents that not only describe his health but also list all the therapeutic and diagnostic procedures applied, and the patient's response to these. Patient charts comprise of Case management, Consent forms, Consultation reports, Contents of patient charts, Core measures, Critical pathways, Flow sheets, Graphic record, History and physical examination form, Kardex records, Laboratory tests record, Medication administration record (MAR), Nurses' notes, Nursing care plans, Other diagnostic reports, Patient education record, Physician's order form, PRN or Unscheduled medication record, Progress notes, and Summary sheet.

Safety

Medication errors may result in the failure of completion of a planned action as intended. Medication errors could be prescribing errors, dispensing errors, transcription errors, administration errors, order communication errors, and monitoring errors. Prescribing errors may result from suboptimal decisions with regards to drug therapy, incorrect dosage, prescription of unauthorized drugs or prescription of a drug for a patient with known intolerability or allergy.

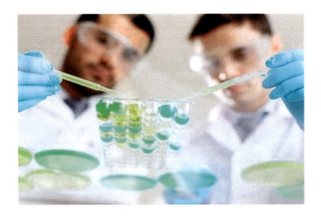

Dispensing errors may result when a wrong dose or drug is sent or a wrong formulation or dosage is ordered. Transcription errors result from misinterpreted order regarding a medication or misunderstanding of directions, usage of unapproved abbreviations and illegible handwriting. Administration errors may involve giving an incorrect dosage, missed dose or extra dose, wrong timing of drug administration or incorrect technique or route of administration. Monitoring related errors include improper monitoring, improper assessments of response to drug, and improper patient education regarding the process.

In order to ensure medication safety, some basic principles can be followed. These include the use of CPOE or other technology, use of bar-code for determining status of drug administration and the use of smart pumps to ensure controlled drug administration. Checklists should be used for high alert drugs. Generic and brand names should be used to avoid errors, especially in the case of drugs whose names sound similar.

High-alert medication should be restricted during the dispensing process away from the readily available floor stock to ensure that they are not mistakenly taken. Verbal orders should be avoided for high-alert medications. The drug dosing infusion charts and concentrations should be standardized. Patient Care Technicians administering medications should perform double checks before administration.

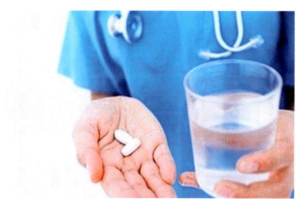

The patient's current orders of medications should be compared with all the other medications he is taking to avoid errors of duplication, omission, drug interactions and dosage. This kind of medication reconciliation is a five-step procedure beginning with the development of a list of the currently administered medications, along with a list of previously prescribed medications. The two lists need to be compared and clinical decisions are taken depending on the comparison made. The new list is to be communicated to the patient, caregivers, supervisors and other healthcare professionals. Appropriate judgments are to be made with respect to the type of drug, allergies, dosage, therapeutic intent, contraindication and physical preparation of the drug dosage. If a healthcare professional with the responsibility of administering the drug feels it inappropriate to administer the drug, a notification is to be sent to the prescriber immediately along with an explanation for the decision taken.

Medication Administration

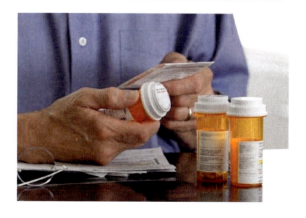

There are six rights of medication administration. These are right medication, right dose, right route, right time, right patient and right documentation.

According to the right to right drug, it is crucial to compare the spelling and concentration of the medication prescribed with the drug profile and medication container before administering it.

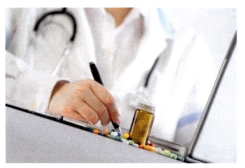

As per the right to right dosage, it is the responsibility of the medication administrator to double check and confirm the supplied medication matches the ordered dosage and is calculated accurately. The dosage should be confirmed to be appropriate for the patient. He should also pay attention if the patient has any concerns or questions regarding the shape, color or size of the medication.

The medication needs to be administered at the right time. While scheduling the time of drug administration, standardized times, time abbreviations, etc. need to be assessed in order to ensure the maintenance of blood levels, enable maximum absorption of drug and other such factors.

While administering a drug to a patient, the name of the patient on the order or medication card should be cross checked with the name on the bracelet. The patient should also be checked for allergies.

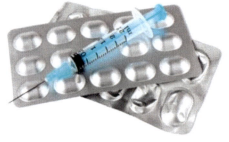

The right route of drug administration is highly crucial in order to ensure the therapeutic efficiency and safety of a drug. The administration of a drug though the IV route delivers it into the blood stream directly. It results in the fastest onset and so, has the highest risk of potential adverse effects. The next fastest absorption occurs upon administration via the intramuscular route depending upon the blood supply availability. However, this route of administration could be painful for the patient. The third fastest route is the subcutaneous route followed by the oral route.

The oral route could be as fast as the intramuscular route depending on the dose form and type of medication, and also on the basis of whether food is present in the stomach of the patient. The oral route is safe for medication administration if a patient is able to swallow and is in a conscious state. The rectal route is to be avoided whenever possible as it causes mucosal tissue irritation and also because its absorption rates are erratic. Right documentation is another critical requirement during drug administration. The chart and reports should cover the date and time of medication administration, name of drug, route, dosage and the site of the administration of the medication. An incident report regarding an error should mention the date, time of ordering of drug, the name of the drug, route and the dosage. Therapeutic response and adverse effects should be noted.

Different Routes of Medication Administration

The route of drug administration is determined based on the properties of the drug, for instance its solubility and ionization, and by the desired therapeutic action (Harvey, 2008). The major routes of drug administration as described by Harvey (2008) are discussed as follows:

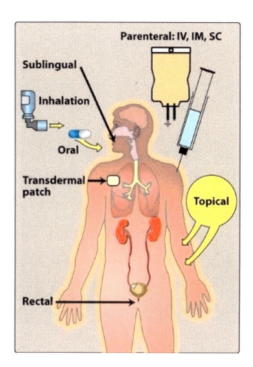

Figure 1: Common routes of administration of medications.

Enteral Route (Oral and Sublingual)

The enteral route of drug administration is the administration of a medication through the mouth, which is the most common, safest, economical and convenient mode. Administration of a medication through the mouth involves swallowing or placing it under the tongue (sublingual). The oral mode of drug administration has many advantages.

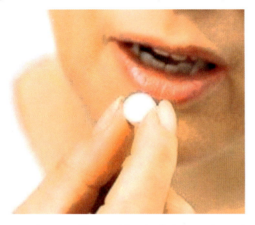

These can be easily self-administered and pose a low systemic infection risk as compared to the parenteral route, which may have complicated the treatment. Overdose or toxicity resulting from oral administration can be easily reversed through appropriate antidotes such as the use of activated charcoal. However, the pathways associated with oral drug absorption are complicated and the low pH in stomach may also result in drug inactivation.

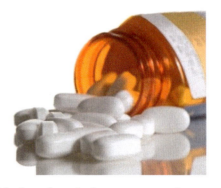

Many kinds of oral drug preparations exist, which include enteric coated preparations and extended release preparations. Enteric coated preparations have an enteric coating which is a chemical envelop that is not affected by the action of enzymes and fluids in the stomach. It dissolves in the upper intestine. This preparation is useful for acid unstable drugs such as omeprazole. Enteric coated drugs are resistant to stomach acid and deliver them in the intestine which is less acidic. Drugs such as aspirin that irritate the stomach can also be coated with a substance that dissolves only in the small intestine to protect the stomach and prevent irritability.

Extended release preparations of medications have special ingredients or coatings that control the speed of drug release from the pill. These have a long duration of action which may be required to improve compliance of patients as the medication need not be taken often. These medications maintain their concentrations within an acceptable therapeutic range for a long time, unlike the immediate release forms of drugs whose plasma concentrations generally have larger troughs and peaks. Extended release dosage preparation is suitable for drugs that have short half-lives.

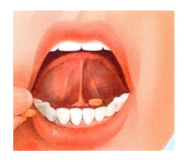

Administration through the sublingual route requires placement of drug under the tongue to facilitate diffusion of the drug into the capillary network and subsequently into the systemic circulation. The advantages of this route are that it facilitates rapid absorption, is easy to administer, has a low incidence of infection, bypasses the gastrointestinal environment which is harsh, and avoids the first-pass metabolism. Another route is the buccal route where the medication is placed between the gum and cheek. This is similar to the sublingual route of medication administration.

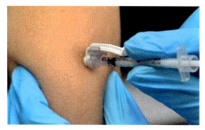

Parenteral Route (Intravenous IV, Intramuscular IM, Subcutaneous SC)

The parenteral route of drug administration introduces drugs into the body's systemic circulation against its barrier defenses. This route of administration is suitable for drugs that are poorly absorbed through the gastrointestinal tract and for agents that are unstable in it. It is also useful for treatment of patients who are unconscious and in whom a rapid onset of action is required. Parenteral route of administration has the highest bioavailability and are not subject to the harsh gastrointestinal environment or the first-pass metabolism. It offers most control over the actual dosage of the delivered drug. This mode of administration is irreversible and could induce fear, pain, infections and local tissue damage. The major parenteral routes include intravascular (IV), which could be intra-arterial or intravenous, intramuscular (IM) or subcutaneous (SC). Each of these routes has its own advantages and disadvantages.

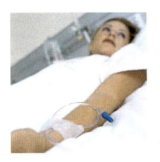

The most common parenteral route of medication administration is IV. In case of drugs that cannot be absorbed orally, such as atracurium, a neuromuscular blocker, there is often no choice other than IV.

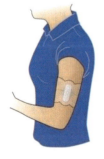 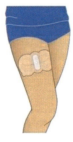

This mode of drug delivery enables a rapid effect and offers the maximum degree of control over the drug's circulating levels. When the drug is injected as bolus, the entire drug is immediately delivered into the systemic circulation. Through IV infusion, the same dose can be administered over a longer time because of which the peak in plasma concentration decreases and the drug is present in the circulation over a longer period of time. IV injection is suitable while administering medications that cause irritation through other routes as the blood dilutes them rapidly. However, injected drugs cannot be recalled using strategies such as activated charcoal unlike those that are administered via the gastrointestinal tract.

Another disadvantage of IV injection is that it may inadvertently introduce infectious agents such as bacteria through contamination, and it may also precipitate the constituents of blood. It may also induce hemolysis and result in other adverse effects due to a very rapid delivery of high drug concentrations into the tissues and plasma. Patients administered through this route need to be monitored carefully for adverse drug reactions so that careful control of the rate of infusion can be carried out.

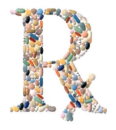

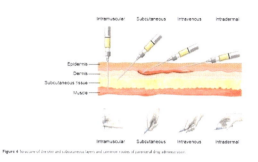

Figure 4 Structure of the skin and subcutaneous layers and common routes of parenteral drug administration.

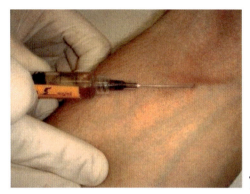 The IM route of drug administration involves the use of an aqueous solution that facilitates rapid absorption. Specialized depot preparations can be used when slow absorption is required. Depot preparations use a nonaqueous vehicle containing a suspension of the drug. The drug precipitates at injection site in the muscle as the vehicle diffuses out. The drug slowly dissolves and a sustained dosage is provided for an extended time period. Some drugs administered through this mode include medroxyprogesterone (depot) and haloperidol (sustained-release).

Subcutaneous route of medication administration is slightly slower than the IV route and absorption is through diffusion. It minimizes the risk of thrombosis and hemolysis that has a greater frequency of occurrence when the route of administration is IV injection. The SC route is not used for drugs that result in tissue irritation, because it may result in necrosis and pain. An example is that of epinephrine, minute amounts of which are combined with a subcutaneously administered drug to confine its area of action. Other examples include etonogestrel.

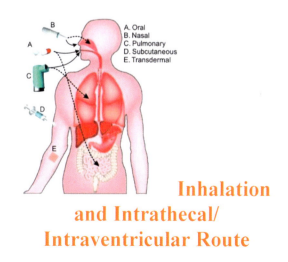

Inhalation and Intrathecal/ Intraventricular Route

Drugs can also be administered through inhalation, both nasal and oral. This route enables rapid drug delivery across mucous membranes of pulmonary epithelium and the respiratory tract, which have a large surface area. The effect of this route is as rapid as IV injection and it is used for gaseous drugs such as certain anesthetics that can be dispersed using an aerosol.

Administration through oral inhalation is highly effective for patients having respiratory disorders such as asthma as the drug is directly delivered to the site of action. This route minimizes side effects. Some of the drugs that are administered via this route include albuterol, a bronchodilator and fluticasone, a corticosteroid.

The nasal inhalation route of administration involves delivery via the nose using nasal sprays. Nasal decongestants like oxymetazoline are administered through this route. Another route is the intrathecal/intraventricular route. This route is used to deliver drugs directly into the cerebrospinal fluid because the blood-brain barrier delays drug absorption into the central nervous system.

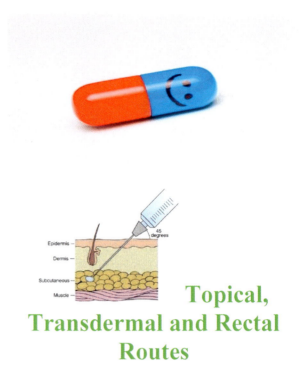

Topical, Transdermal and Rectal Routes

Some drugs are applied topically for a local effect. Examples include clotrimazole, a cream that is applied directly on the skin for treating dermatophytosis.

The transdermal route of administration is used when systemic effects are desired by applying drugs on the skin, usually using a transdermal patch.

This route is used when a sustained delivery of drugs is required. For instance, scopolamine, an antiemetic is administered using a transdermal patch. The rectal route of administration of medication is employed to prevent destruction of drugs by intestinal enzymes or due to fluids or low pH in the stomach. It also minimizes the liver biotransformation of drugs. This route is also suitable if a drug causes vomiting through oral ingestion, if a patient is already in the condition of vomiting, or if he is not conscious for oral administration. It is commonly used for the administration of antiemetics.

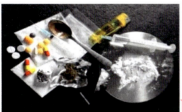

Drugs Affecting Various Systems of the Human Body

Medications target different systems of the human body and are classified accordingly. Some important drug categories that act on the various systems are discussed here (Rosenfeld and Loose, 2014; Aehlert and Vroman, 2011):

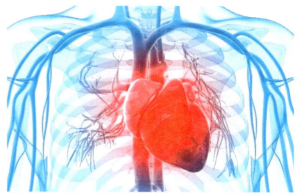

Drugs Affecting the Cardiovascular System

Drugs that are used for the treatment of congestive heart failure (CHF) include angiotensin-converting enzyme (ACE) inhibitors such as Captopril and Enalapril, and angiotensin receptor blockers (ARBs) such as Valsartan. Other drugs used for the treatment of CHF are cardiac glycosides and inotropic agents such as milrinone. Diuretics and vasodilators are also used. Antiarrhythmic drugs used for treatment of Arrhythmias include Quinidine and Procainamide.

Antianginal agents include nitrates and nitirites, β-Adrenoceptor antagonists and Calcium channel-blocking agents (CCB) such as Nifedipine. Antihypertensive drugs include β-Adrenoceptor antagonists such as Propranolol and α-Adrenoceptor antagonists such as Labetalol. Renin inhibitors such as

Aliskiren, antihypertensive agents such as hydralazine, and specialized vasodilators such as Ambrisentan are some of the other drugs that affect the cardiovascular system.

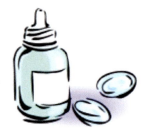

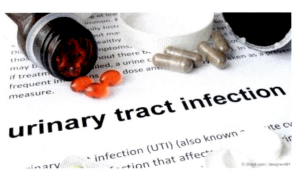

Drugs Affecting the Urinary System

Some of the drugs that affect the urinary system include diuretics such as Thiazide diuretics, Thiazide-like drugs such as chlorthalidone and loop diuretics such as furosemide. Carbonic anhydrase inhibitors used for treatment of glaucoma are also used for enhancing the renal secretion of cysteine and uric acid. Agents that influence the excretion of water include osmotic agents like mannitol and urea. Nondiuretic inhibitors, Uricosuric agents and other agents such as Allopurinol are also employed in treatment of disorders related to the urinary system.

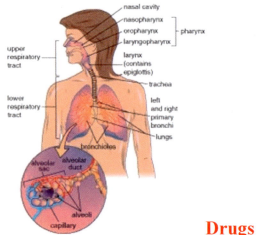

Drugs Affecting the Respiratory System

Drugs affecting the respiratory system include decongestants, antitussives, expectorants, antihistamines, and mucolytics. Antitussives used for controlling nonproductive cough include codeine, benzonatate and Dextromethorphan. Other drugs that affect the respiratory system include topical nasal decongestants such as Ephedrine, oral decongestants, topical nasal steroids such as Flunisolide, antihistamines such as Diphenhydramine, expectorants such as Guaifenesin and mucolytics such as acetylcysteine.

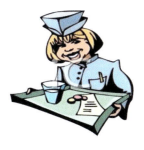

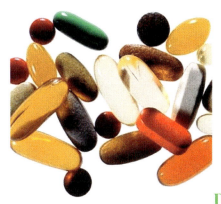

Drugs Affecting the Digestive System, Vitamins, and Minerals

Drugs affecting the digestive system include those that are used for peptic ulcers and those that are used to modulate gastroentric functions. Anti-ulcer drugs include antacids, drugs such as muscarinic receptor antagonists, H2 receptor antagonists, proton pump inhibitors that inhibit secretion of gastric acid, mucosal protective drugs and antimicrobial drugs. Common antacids include Aluminium hydroxide and Magnesium trisilicate. Muscarinic receptor antagonists include Atropine and Telenzepine. H2 receptor antagonists include Ranitidine, proton pump inhibitors include Omeprazole. Mucosal protective drugs include Misoprostol and Marzulene. Antimicrobial drugs include Tetracycline and Amoxicillin. Modulator drugs influencing gastroenteric functions include antiemetic (Diphenhydramine, Scopolamine, etc.) and prokinetic drugs (Metoclopramide, Domperidone, etc.), laxatives (Phenolphthalein, Magnesium sulfate, etc.) and diarrhea treating drugs (Diphenoxylate, Tannalbin, etc.).

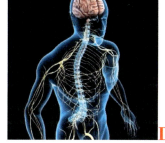

Drugs Affecting the Central Nervous System (CNS)

Drugs affecting the CNS include depressants such as sedatives and hypnotics, which include Barbiturates, Benzodiazepines, etc. Sedative-hypnotic drugs include flurazepam, which is long acting, and estazolam, which is short acting. Anxiolytic (anxiety relieving) drugs include alprazolam, lorazepam, diazepam and chloridiazepoxide.

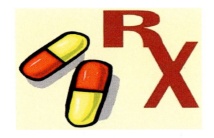

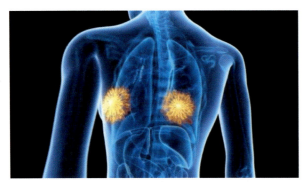

Drugs Affecting the Musculoskeletal System

These include uricosuric drugs such as colchicine, indomethacin (a non-steroidal antiinflammatry drug, and allopurinol). Colchicine is used for relieving the symptoms of gout. It is an alkaloid that suppresses the initial immune reaction responsible for pain.

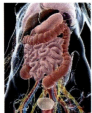

Drugs Affecting the Endocrine System

Drugs affecting the pituitary gland include octreotide, somatrem and sermorelin for the anterior pituitary gland and vasopressin and desmopressin for the posterior pituitary gland. Drugs affecting the thyroid and parathyroid are calciferol, plicamycin, liotrix and levothyroxine. In addition, certain steroids and corticosteroids influence the adrenal cortex. These include hydrocortisone, dexamethasone, hydrocortisone sodium succinate and fludrocortisone.

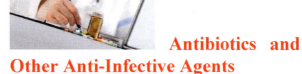

Antibiotics and Other Anti-Infective Agents

These include aerosolized anti-infective agents such as Pentamidine isethionate, Ribavirin, and Zanamivir; aerosolized antibiotics, non-aerosolized anti-infective agents such as cell wall affecting agents like Penicillins, Bacitracin, Vancomycin, protein synthesis inhibiting agents like Chloramphenicol, Streptomycin, Kanamycin, Lincomycin, Gentamicin, and Aminoglycosides and nucleic acid synthesis inhibiting agents like Mitomycin, Rifampicin and Actinomycin. Antibiotics are classified as bactericidal (Cephalosporins,

Streptomycin, Cycloserine, Penicillins, Polymyxins, Kanamycin) and bacteriostatic (Tetracyclines, Chloramphenicol, Erythromycin). They are also classified alternatively as broad spectrum (Chloramphenicol, Cephalosporins, Ampicillin, Kanamycin) and narrow spectrum (Erythromycin, Polymyxin B, Penicillin).

Synthetic (nonantibiotic) anti-infective agents include Sulfonamides (Sulfamethoxazole, Sulfisoxazole, Sulfamethizole, Sulfacytine), Trimethoprim-Sulfamethoxazole and Nitrofurantoin. Antifungal agents include Nystatin, Amphotericin B and Griseofulvin. Antituberculosis agents include Streptomycin, Pyrazinamide, Rifampin, Isoniazid and Ethambutol. Antiviral agents include Acyclovir, Didanosine, Ganciclovir, Idoxuridine, Rimantadine and Vidarabine.

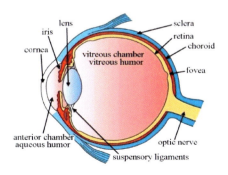

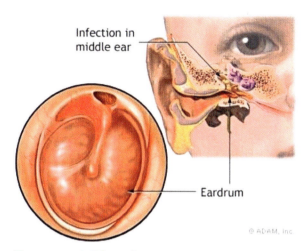

Drugs Affecting the Eye and Ear

Drugs applied to the eye may have many purposes which include treatment of a medical condition, prevention of eye infection and for the enhancement of eye examination. Some of the drugs affecting the eye include antiglaucoma agents, cycloplegic and mydriatic agents, topical anesthetic agents, anti-infective agents, anti-inflammatory agents, and other ophthalmic preparations. Anti-glaucoma agents used to treat glaucoma include beta blockers such as betaxolol and timolol, carbonic anhydrase inhibitors such as acetazolamide, prostaglandin analogs such as latanoprost, sympathomimetics such as brimonidine and other agents such as pilocarpine. Cycloplegic and mydriatic agents are administered to dilate the pupil and to treat inflammation and pain. Examples of these agents include cyclopentolate hydrochloride, epinephrine, homatropine ophthalmic solution, and atropine ophthalmic solution. Topical anesthetic agents are used as local anesthetics for pain reduction. These include proparacaine HCL and tetracocaine HCL. Other preparations used for ophthalmic administration include lubricants and artificial tears. Drugs affecting the ear include anti-inflammatory agents, antibiotics and wax buildup suppressing agents. Topical otic preparatons such as drops usually contain antibiotics.

Patient Care Procedures

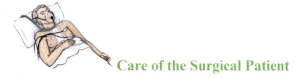

Care of the Surgical Patient

A. Perform tasks from pre-operative checklist
   1. Showering, bathing
   2. Enemas - per hospital policy
   3. Nonsterile douche - per hospital policy
   4. Shave prep
   5. Hospital gown
   6. NPO after midnight or as ordered by physician
   7. Vital signs
   8. Remove dentures, if ordered.
   9. Remove prostheses (i.e., hearing aids, glasses, contact lenses, splints, braces, artificial parts).
   10. Remove jewelry, hair pins, makeup.
   11. Tape wedding rings, if allowed.
   12. Assure security of any items of value (i.e., give jewelry to family member with patient's permission).
   13. Have patient empty bladder. Drain Foley if present. Record output.
   14. Notify medication nurse when patient is ready.
   15. Provide for safe environment after pre-operative medication (i.e., side rails up, safety belt fastened on gurney, call light in reach).

B. **Identify nurse assistant's role in pre-operational checklist**
C. **Document on the preoperative checklist**

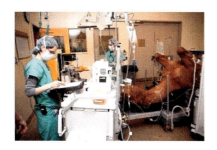

Nurse assistant's responsibilities while the patient is in surgery.

A. **Prepare the room:**
   1. Surgical bed
   2. Emesis basin
   3. Facial tissue
   4. Vital sign equipment
   5. IV pole
   6. Incontinent pads.
B. **Collect additional equipment as ordered**
   1. O_2 equipment
   2. Pulse Oximeter
   3. Suction

Patient care measures provided in the post-operative phase.

A. **Post-operative checks**
   1. Note time of return.
   2. Note level of consciousness.
   3. Check dressings for location and condition (dryness).
   4. Observe incisions, report any drainage, redness or swelling (assessing and changing the dressing is the responsibility of the licensed nurse).
   5. Check IV for location and observe site for redness, swelling, warmth or drainage.
   6. Observe to see that IV is dripping and tubing not kinked.

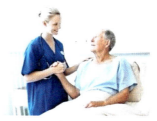

B. **Post-operative care measures**
   1. Assist in transfer from gurney to bed.
   2. Vital signs
      a. Be aware of changes in vital signs that signal hemorrhage, i.e., decreasing blood pressure and increasing pulse.
      b. Elevated temperature may signal infection.
      c. Report abnormalities to licensed personnel promptly.
      d. Pulse oximetry

3. **Observations**
   a. Comfort: degree of pain or other discomfort
   b. Safety: side rails, call light within reach
   c. Equipment: report if disconnected or malfunctioning
   d. Changes in behavior: confusion, disorientation, agitation

e. Changes in skin color: pallor, gray, blue-tinged
f. Nausea, vomiting
g. Bowel activity, passing gas

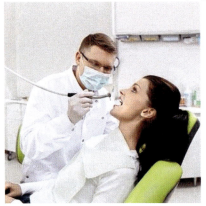

C. **Care measures to prevent complications**
1. Encourage
   a. Turn, cough and deep breathing
   b. Incentive spirometer
   c. Leg exercises
2. Apply TED hose and sequential compression de-vices, if ordered.
3. Reposition at least every 2 hours to prevent hypo-static pneumonia.
4. Apply binders, if ordered.
5. Assist with dangling and initial ambulation, as ordered
6. Review Hazards of Immobility and Role of the Nurse Assistant.

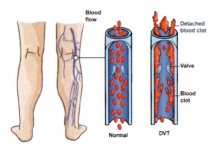

D. **Complications of Immobility: Deep Vein Thrombosis (DVT) – blood clot in lower extremity**

1. **General Information**
   a. Deep vein thrombus (DVT) or blood clot occurs in pelvic veins or in deep veins of the lower extremities in post-operative patients. The incidence of DVT varies between 10% and 40% depending upon how serious the surgery is and how many other medical problems the patient has.
   b. DVT is most common following hip surgery, then prostate surgery and general thoracic or abdominal surgery.
   c. Blood clots located above the knee are considered the major source of pulmonary emboli (a blood clot that dislodges from the vein wall and travels to the lungs, causing death of lung tissue).

2. Causes
   a. Pooling of blood in lower extremities (venous stasis)
   b. Inactivity and immobility
   c. Some medical conditions (stroke, heart attack, congestive heart failure)
   d. Obesity
   e. Varicose veins
   f. Surgery and anesthesia
   g. Age, particularly over 65 years
   h. Damage to or stretching of blood vessels during surgery or trauma
   i. Central venous catheters, pacemaker wires
   j. Previous DVT
   k. Increased tendency of blood to clot (some diseases like cancer, blood diseases, protein deficiency in malnourishment, dehydration)
   l. Oral contraceptives and estrogen replacement
   m. Smoking

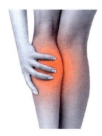

3. Symptoms of DVT
   a. Often have no symptoms
   b. Pain or cramp in the calf or thigh, progressing to painful swelling of entire leg
   c. Slight fever, chills, perspiration (diaphoresis), generalized feeling of discomfort
   d. Painful tenderness over inner thigh

4. Prevention
   a. Increased activity, early ambulation after surgery, frequent and proper repositioning
   b. Range of motion
   c. Anti-embolic stockings (TED hose)
   d. Purpose of anti-embolic stockings
      1) To help prevent formation of blood clots
      2) To promote increased blood flow in the legs by compression of deep veins
      3) To improve venous return from the legs to the heart maintenance of anti-embolic stockings
      4) Properly sized stockings need to be removed daily during bathing to inspect condition of skin. Do not leave off more than 30 minutes.

5) Wash stockings every 2 to 3 days to remove bodily secretions.
6) For patient's information at home, the stockings can usually be machine washed on delicate and machine dried on low for 15 to 20 minutes.
7) With correct care stockings last 3 to 4 months.
8) Do not use ointments on the leg when using anti-embolic stockings.
e. Sequential compressions sleeves or devices
f. Adequate fluids
g. Avoid dependent positioning of lower extremities (elevate legs when up in chair, avoid knee gatch when in bed).
h. Doctor may order anticoagulants for licensed nurse to administer; observe for signs of bleeding or bruising.
i. Observe for pain in calf, fever or chills, painful swelling of leg, tenderness over inner thigh.
j. Report any shortness of breath or chest pain immediately to the licensed nurse.

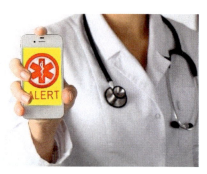

E. Nursing Alert

1. *A complaint of slight soreness of the calf is never ignored. Blood clots in the calf or thigh can break loose and travel to the lungs (pulmonary embolism). This is life threatening.*
2. *Close observation of patients and attention to their complaints of pain or discomfort is very important.*
3. *Report this to the licensed nurse.*
4. *Never rub or massage the lower legs.*

SEQUENTIAL COMPRESSION DEVICES

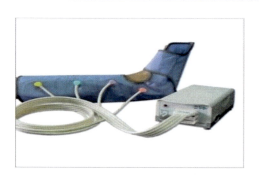

Several types of devices are available that supply intermittent compression over the lower leg, thigh or foot. Each device aids in the return of venous blood and helps prevent deep vein thrombosis and pulmonary embolism. They are usually used in addition to anti-embolic stockings.

The typical type of sequential compression device consists of a vinyl or plastic sleeve that fits over the foot, lower leg or thigh. It may come as a tube or as a wrap style that fastens with Velcro. It is attached to a control unit that is placed on the floor under the bed.

The control unit has a small pump that inflates and deflates channels in the sleeve to provide increasing and decreasing pressure. Connecting tubing attaches to the sleeve and to the control unit completing a closed system. The pressure can be adjusted according to facility policy or as ordered by the physician.

The device should be removed at least twice daily for 20 to 30 minutes to allow for ambulation, bathing and inspection of the skin. Sequential compression devices are usually worn at least 3 days after surgery or until the patient is up and ambulating regularly or as long as the doctor orders.

EQUIPMENT:

1. Sequential compression sleeves
2. Connectors
3. Control unit

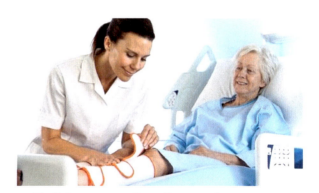

Safely cares for the patient on a sequential compression device

1. Wash hands, identify patient, introduce self, explain procedure and provide for privacy.
2. Position patient, exposing one leg at a time for application of sequential sleeve.

3. Align leg on the open sleeve according to instructions included in package.
4. Wrap the sleeve securely around the patient's leg and fasten the Velcro tabs, thigh section first. Make sure that no wrinkles are in the plastic of the sleeve and that at least two fingers can be inserted between the patient's leg and the sleeve.
5. Make sure the control unit is turned off.
6. Attach the connector on the sleeve to the correct end of the connector tubing. Check carefully to be certain there are no kinks or twists in the tubing.
7. Attach the other end of the connector tubing to the control unit.
8. Turn the power on and adjust or monitor the pressure according to your facility's policy.
9. Remain with the patient for at least a complete cycle to monitor comfort and the functioning of the unit.
10. Sleeves should be removed if the patient experiences numbness, tingling or leg pain. Notify licensed nurse if any of these symptoms occur.
11. Document time of application, type of device, condition of skin and comfort of patient.

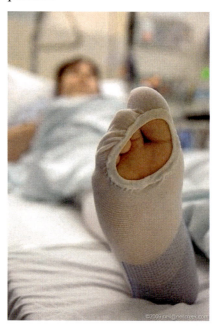

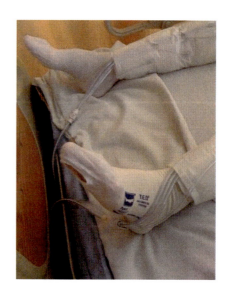

PRECAUTIONS:

1. Do not apply to any patient experiencing skin rash or poor circulation evidenced by bluish-red coloring of lower legs and feet, sores on lower legs or feet, severe edema or leg pain, edema of the lungs from congestive heart failure.
2. Make sure that connectors and sleeves are properly applied.
3. Monitor the patient's condition frequently, according to facility policy.

SINGLE LEG APPLICATION:

1. Most brands of sequential compression devices can be used on only one leg, if necessary.
2. The unused sleeve is kept in the plastic wrapper and attached to the second sleeve connector.
3. The compression action of the pump will not work unless there is a closed system. By keeping the unused sleeve folded in the wrapper, the system will be able to reach the proper compression.

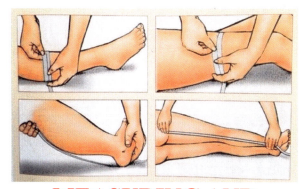

MEASURING AND APPLICATION OF ANTI-EMBOLIC STOCKINGS

EQUIPMENT:

1. Tape measure (new one for each patient)
2. Scratch pad, order form or requisition form from Central Supply
3. Anti-embolic stockings (TED stockings or other brands)

CRITERIA:

Correctly measures and applies anti-embolic stockings

A. Thigh length
1. Measure upper thigh circumference at gluteal furrow.
2. Measure calf circumference at widest area.
3. Measure length from gluteal furrow to base of heel.

4. Consult sizing chart from Central Supply or TED stockings order pad, if available.
    - TED thigh length with belt stocking fit a thigh circumference of up to 32 inches.
    - TED thigh length stocking fit a maximum thigh circumference of 25 inches.

B. Knee length

1. Measure calf circumference at widest area.
2. Measure length from bend of knee to base of heel.

C. Medicare usually covers two pair to insure that compression goes uninterrupted during laundering care. Check with the RN to see if one or two pair should be ordered.

D. Different brands of anti-embolic elastic stockings are available. Each pair will have a large round hole in the toe to check for circulation. In some brands the hole will be on top of the toes and some will have the hole open under the toes.

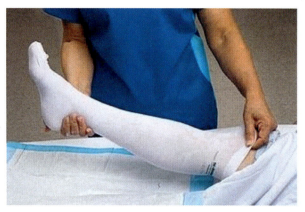

APPLICATION OF ANTI-EMBOLIC STOCKINGS:

1. Obtain correct size of anti-embolic stockings.
2. Wash hands, identify patient, introduce self, explain procedure and provide for privacy.
3. With patient lying down, expose one leg at a time for application of stocking.
4. Insert hand into stocking as far as the heel pocket.
5. Grasp center of heel pocket and turn stocking inside out to heel area.
6. Position stocking over foot and heel. Be sure patient's heel is centered in heel pocket.
7. Pull a few inches of the stocking up around the ankle and calf.
8. Continue pulling the stocking up the leg. If there is a change in the sheerness of the stocking material, it should fall between 1" to 2" below the bend of the knee.

9. As thigh portion of the stocking is applied, start rotating stocking inward so gusset is centered over femoral artery. Gusset is placed slightly towards the inside of the leg. When using thigh length stockings, the top band rests in the gluteal furrow.
10. Smooth out wrinkles.
11. Align inspection toe to fall at base of toes either on the top or underneath, depending on brand.
12. Instruct patient on proper positioning of stockings to insure that he/she will not reposition the stockings incorrectly.
13. Repeat procedure on opposite leg.
14. Wash hands.
15. Report procedure and document size and style of stocking applied.
16. Document when stockings are removed along with condition of skin.
17. Report any tenderness in calves, thighs or toes.

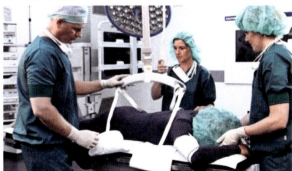

TURNING A SURGICAL PATIENT

EQUIPMENT:

1. Pillows
2. Lift sheet

CRITERIA:

Safely turns a surgical patient

Instruct patient in splinting incision for comfort.

1. Obtain patient activity orders from licensed nurse.
2. Instruct patient in splinting incision for comfort.
3. Make sure that bed wheels are locked, curtains are pulled around bed for privacy and bed is raised to highest level for good body mechanics.
4. Lower head of bed if patient's condition allows.
5. Using good body mechanics, turn patient.
6. Position patient for comfort and in good body alignment.
   a. Place pillow under head.
   b. Position a pillow against back for support.

c. Place a pillow in front of the bottom leg and place the top leg on top of the pillow in a flexed position.
d. Check lower shoulder to make sure it is not squeezed in an abnormal position. Reach under shoulder and pull forward gently until patient is comfortable.
e. Support upper arm and hand with a pillow for comfort, either in front of the patient or back on the pillow behind the patient.
f. If abdominal incision is pulling, may place pillow under side of abdomen.
7. Place the signal cord within reach; raise side rails, lower bed to lowest position, open curtains around bed.

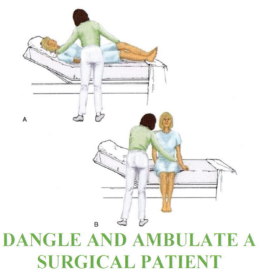

DANGLE AND AMBULATE A SURGICAL PATIENT

CRITERIA:

Safely Dangles and Ambulates a Surgical Patient

1. Check patient's pulse, blood pressure and respirations.
2. Assist patient to side of bed and put on non-slip slippers.
3. Assist patient to pivot and sit at side of bed.
4. Support patient and observe for abnormal signs.
5. Assist patient to put on robe.
6. Apply gait belt if allowed.
7. Assist the patient to stand.
8. Stand at patient's side until steady, holding the gait belt in the middle of the patient's back.
9. Stand slightly behind patient, on weak side, if applicable.
10. Encourage patient to walk with head up, standing erect.
11. Observe for signs of activity intolerance (increased pain, shortness of breath, pallor, diaphoresis).

12. Return patient to bed and make sure patient is safe and comfortable.
13. Report distance patient walked and how well patient tolerated activity to licensed nurse.
14. If patient has an IV, may need two people to assist with ambulation.

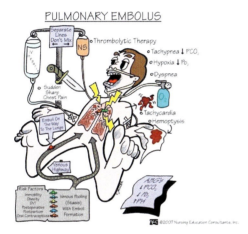

HAZARDS OF IMMOBILITY AND ROLE OF THE NURSE ASSISTANT

1. **Cardiovascular complications -** blood clots, orthostatic hypotension, increased work on the heart
   - Remind patient to do exercises given by the physical and occupational therapist.
   - Encourage intake of adequate fluids to prevent dehydration.
   - Early ambulation as allowed.
   - Proper positioning and avoidance of pressure on blood vessels.
   - Do not massage the calf of the leg.

2. **Respiratory complications** – slow and shallow respirations, pooling of respiratory secretions, hypostatic pneumonia, pulmonary embolism
   - Remind patient to turn, cough, take deep breaths and to use incentive spirometer.
   - Increase activity as soon as allowed by patient's condition and doctor's orders.
   - Encourage fluids as allowed to keep lung secretions thinned.

3. **Gastrointestinal complications –** poor appetite, poor nutrition, constipation, fecal impaction
- Offer adequate fluids.
   - Prevent incontinence by timely offering of the bedpan and early

mobility for access to the bathroom.

- Monitor patient's appetite and ask RN to assess need for a dietician consult.

4. **Urinary system complications –** urinary retention, incontinence, increased risk of kidney stones, urinary tract infections
    - Keep accurate record of intake and output.
    - Observe for pain in the back and blood in the urine.
    - Observe for signs of urinary tract infection: pain with urination, frequent urination of small amounts, feeling the need to urinate all the time, concentrated or cloudy urine.

5. **Musculoskeletal system** complications – muscle wasting and atrophy, stiff joints, decreased balance, loss of endurance, osteoporosis, contractures, foot drop
    - Perform passive ROM exercises for patients who are unable to do them, and instruct patients who are able to do active or active-assistive ROM.
    - Position patients properly in bed, using good body alignment.
    - Remind and reinforce any exercises given to patient by physical or occupational therapists and RN.

6. **Integumentary system complications** – pressure on bony prominences, impaired circulation to skin layers, skin breakdown, pressure ulcers, infections
    - Observe for any sign of redness or sores on the skin.
    - Keep skin clean and dry.
    - Keep bedding free of wrinkles and crumbs.
    - Turn patient at least every 2 hours to reduce pressure on bony prominence

GASTRO-INTESTINAL CARE

Common diseases/disorders of the GI system.

A. Congenital: cleft palate
B. Inflammation: stomatitis, esophagitis, gastro-enteritis, colitis,

    cholecystitis, pancreatitis, hepatitis, cholelithiasis
  C. Ulceration: stomach, duodenum, colon
  D. Hernias: inguinal, umbilical, hiatal, inicisional.
  E. Tumors: benign, malignant
  F. Bowel disorders: distension, diarrhea, constipation, and impaction

Patient preparation for GI diagnostic tests.

  A. **Radiology Testing**
    1. UGI
    2. Small bowel series
    3. Gall bladder series
    4. Barium enema
  B. **Direct Visualization**
    1. Colonoscopy/sigmoidoscopy
    2. Esophagogastroduodenoscopy (EGD)
    3. Gastroscopy
    4. Endoscopy
    5. Swallowing evaluation
    6. Gastric sampling
    7. Ultrasound
  C. **Preparing the patient for diagnostic tests**
    1. NPO for at least eight hours (or as ordered)
    2. Give enemas as ordered.
    3. Laxatives given by licensed nurse as ordered.

Special Diets as Ordered

A. Purpose of enemas: to aid in illumination during x-rays, before surgery, before deliveries, before direct visualization tests, for bowel retraining, to relieve constipation, to expel flatus, to instill medicine.
B. Types of enemas
  1. Cleansing: SSE, TWE, saline, Fleet's phosphosoda.
  2. Retention: medicinal, nutritional, Fleet's oil retention.
  3. Return Flow: Harris flush (HF).
A. Purpose of the sitz bath.
  1. Cleansing
  2. Heat

Healing after perineal/rectal surgery or infant delivery

A. Abnormal signs and symptoms to report to licensed nurse.
  1. Weakness
  2. Rapid, weak pulse
  3. Low blood pressure
  4. Rapid or labored respirations
  5. Fatigue
  6. Dizziness

7. Fainting
8. Bleeding (coffee grounds emesis, black, tarry stools, rectal bleeding)
9. Change in drainage
10. Change in stool

The difference in care measures between hemodialysis and peritoneal dialysis.

A. **Hemodialysis:**
   1. Procedure that filters and cleans waste products from the blood. It is performed by specially trained RNs.
   2. Never take blood pressure in arm with a fistula or shunt

B. **Peritoneal dialysis:**
   1. Removes extra water, waste, and chemicals from body by perfusing sterile solutions through the peritoneal cavity and using the thin membrane that lines the abdominal organs, (peritoneum) as a filter. The dialyzed solution drains out through an abdominal tube.
   2. Reporting abnormal signs and symptoms
      a. Fever, nausea/vomiting
      b. Abdominal pain
      c. Redness around the catheter
      d. Change in vital signs
   3. Special considerations - no ointments or powder around peritoneal catheter.
   4. Prevention of infection
   5. Standard precautions

Reproductive System Care

The common sexually transmitted diseases (STDs).

A. Syphilis
B. Gonorrhea
C. Herpes simplex
D. Venereal warts
E. AIDS
F. **Chlamydia**
   1. Method of transmission:
      a. Mucous membrane to mucous membrane
      b. Mucous membrane to skin
      c. Skin to mucous membrane
   2. Stress nursing considerations: importance of treating all patients

with respect and avoiding judgmental attitude regarding patient's lifestyle.

Care Measures for the Postpartum Patient.

A. Observe vaginal discharge for color/odor
  1. Lochia rubra: dark or bright red 3-4 days
  2. Lochia serosa: pinkish brown 10 days
  3. Lochia alba: whitish 2-6 weeks
B. Report number of pads used
C. Observe perineal area for signs of infection
D. Set up sitz bath
E. Assist mom with breastfeeding
F. Watch for signs of urine retention
G. Report bowel activity
H. Burning on urination
I. Leg pain, tenderness, swelling
J. Sadness or feelings of depression
K. Breast pain, tenderness, swelling

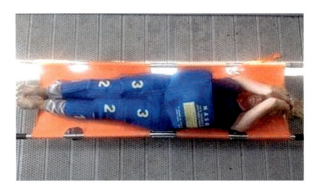

Reportable signs and symptoms of postpartum complications.

A. Fever
B. Abdominal or perineal pain
C. Foul smelling vaginal discharge
D. Bleeding from episiotomy or c-section incision
E. Redness/swelling or drainage from c-section incision
F. Saturating sanitary napkin within one hour of application
G. Red lochia after changed to brown

Post-partum care means care after delivery

REFERENCES

Aehlert, B., & Vroman, R. (2011). *Paramedic Practice Today: Above and Beyond*. Massachusetts: Jones & Bartlett Publishers.

Clayton, B. D. (2012). *Basic Pharmacology for Nurses16: Basic Pharmacology for Nurses*. Missouri: Elsevier Health Sciences.

Durgin, J. M., & Hanan, Z. I. (2004). *Thomson Delmar Learning's Pharmacy Practice for Technicians*. New York: Cengage Learning.

FitzGerald, R. J. (2009). Medication errors: the importance of an accurate drug history. *British Journal of Clinical Pharmacology, 67*(6), 671-675.

Flynn, E. A. (n.d.). *A brief history of medication errors*. Retrieved from http://www.medaccuracy.com/Papers%20and%20Publications/A%20Brief%20History%20of%20Medication%20Errors.pdf.

French, L., & Fordney, M. (2012). *Administrative Medical Assisting*. New York: Cengage Learning.

Harvey, R. (2008). *Lippincott's Illustrated Review: Pharmacology*. Pennsylvania: Lippincott Williams & Wilkins.

Maryland Board of Nursing. (2008, February 27). *Medicine Aides versus Medication Technicians - What's the Difference*. Retrieved from http://www.mbon.org/main.php?v=norm&c=medtech/medaide_vs_medtech.html.

Whitenton, L., & Walker, M. (2013). *MACE Exam Cram: Medication Aide Certification Exam*. Pearson Certification.

Section Two

AN OVERVIEW OF ELECTROCARDIOGRAPH

 INTRODUCTION

The heart is a vital organ of the body. All the blood in the human body is pumped from the heart to different parts of the body. Defects and conditions of the heart are life threatening. The electrocardiogram is a machine that detects the heart's electrical activity and is used to assist in diagnosis. Electrocardiogram technologists are being trained to work with the physicians and cardiologist, especially as cardiovascular problems are on the increase (Hummel et al, 1999, p. 34). This study guide will discuss the human heart, its conduction system, the electrocardiogram machine, heart electrophysiology and how it works. A simple guide to interpretation of EKG Strips will also be provided.

 DUTIES OF AN EKG TECHNICIAN

The EKG technician needs a knowledge of basic medical equipment operation as well as the techniques to monitor a patient's heart electrical activity. Medical equipment used includes the electrocardiogram whose data inform cardiologists and physicians' decision on arriving at the appropriate diagnosis. Electrocardiogram technician are often trained while working by the cardiologists or electrocardiogram supervisor.

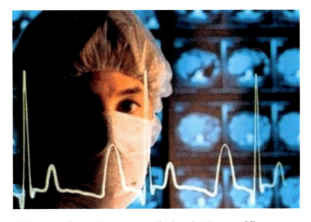

While in the cardiologist's office or laboratory, an EKG technician task involves moving patients and equipment to ensure smooth procedure and patient comfortability. Their work involves dealing with ill and ambulatory patients with heart conditions. When conducting an electrograph, the technician attaches electrodes to the patient at the appropriate positions and operates the machine to generate the heart electrical activity. The physician or the cardiologist conducts the reading for the electrocardiogram machine which is used to analyze the condition of the patient's heart.

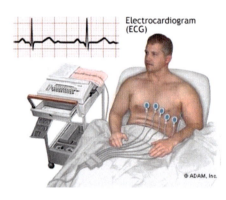

The Electrocardiogram technician can also be involved in stress testing. The electrocardiogram technician attaches electrodes to the patient's heart appropriately to connect the patient to the electrocardiogram machine. While the patient is exercising on the treadmill, the EKG technician takes a baseline reading. The patient is subjected to low speed and high speed on the treadmill to provide reading at diversified physical force.

The technician with advanced training can conduct Holter monitoring. This entails connecting an electrocardiogram to the patient and having them proceed with their daily routine. The holter monitor is removed after a complete day. Then, the electrocardiogram technician uses a scanner to produce the data recorded in the electrocardiogram machine.

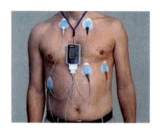

A patient with a holter monitor

GENERAL ANATOMY OF THE HEART

The human heart is composed of cardiac muscles (made up of myocardial cells) to form an organ that is cone shaped. Myocardial tissue forms a large portion of the heart. Endothelium refers to the inner part of the heart. The heart can be compared to be the size of the fist. The heart beats to bring about the flow of blood in the body. It expands and contracts numerous times. It is found between the right and left lungs, enclosed between the lungs and the ribcage and to the left side of the sternum (breast bone). The size of the heart is dependent on the size and age of the individual. The condition of the heart can affect its size.

LAYERS OF THE HEART

- *Endocardium* - the innermost layer of the heart. It forms the lining and folds back onto itself to form the four valves. It is in this layer that the conduction system is found.
- *Myocardium* - the middle and contractile layer of the heart. It is made up of striated muscle fibers interspersed with intercalated disks.
- *Epicardium* – the outermost layer of the heart. It is actually the inner (visceral) layer of the pericardium.

The heart is enclosed by a double layer of protective and connective tissue known as the pericardium. Fibrous pericardium is found on the outside and protects the heart from surrounding organs. The pericardium protects large blood vessels. Fibrous pericardium is attached to some body parts that include spinal column and diaphragm by ligaments. Serous pericardium holds fast to hearts surface and is therefore attached to heart muscles. Between the fibrous pericardium and serous pericardium is pericardial fluid that reduces the friction that results from the contraction of the heart (Gomella 2006, p. 347).

1. **Internal Heart Structure**

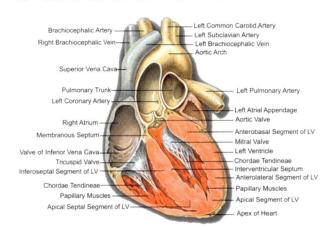

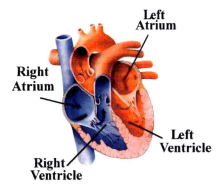

The heart consists of **four chambers**. The right atrium (auricles), left atrium, right ventricle and left ventricle. The septum separates the right chambers from the left chambers. The Atria (plural of atrium) have less muscular walls than the ventricles. The left side of the heart contains oxygenated blood while the right

63

side of the heart receives deoxygenated blood.

Right Atrium – receives deoxygenated blood returning to the heart from the body via the superior vena cava which carries blood from the upper body; and the inferior vena cava which carries blood from the lower body.

Right ventricle – receives deoxygenated blood from the right atrium which it pumps to the lungs for oxygenation through the pulmonary artery (trunk) to the right and left pulmonary arteries.

The *pulmonary arteries* are the only arteries in the body that carry deoxygenated blood.

Left atrium – receives oxygenated blood returning from the lungs via the right and left pulmonary veins.

The *pulmonary veins* are the only veins in the body that carry oxygenated blood.

Left ventricle – receives the oxygenated blood from the left atrium and pumps it to the body through the aorta, the largest artery of the body.

The heart is actually a two-sided pump separated by a septum. The upper chambers consist of the right and left atria (singular: atrium); the lower chambers are the right and left ventricles. The chambers pump simultaneously – both atria contract together then the two ventricles. Picture it as if you have a balloon in your hands, you squeeze the top portion to increase the lower portion of the balloon. After that you squeeze the lower portion of the balloon to increase air in the top portion. The top portion you squeezed represents the atria, while the lower portion represents the ventricles.

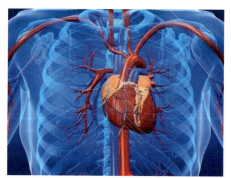

The heart is made up of **valves** that regulate blood flow. The tricuspid valve is responsible for regulating blood flow between the right atrium and right ventricle. The pulmonary valve regulate blood flow between the right ventricle and the pulmonary artery. Pulmonary artery transport blood to lungs for oxygenation. The Mitral valve (also known as bicuspid valve) is located between the left ventricle and the left atrium. Aortic valve allows oxygenated blood from left ventricle into the aorta, from where it flows back into the body. The Aorta is the largest artery in the body.

The purpose of the heart valves is to prevent backflow of blood thereby assuring uni-directional flow through the heart. See names of valves below: The *atrioventricular* valves (AV): so-called because they are located between the atria and ventricles.

a.) Tricuspid valve – located between the right atrium and the right ventricle. As the name connotes, it has three cusps.

b.) Mitral valve – located between the left atrium and the left ventricle. It has two cusps and it also called the bicuspid valve.

The *semilunar* valves: called semilunar because they have half-moon shaped cusps

a.) Pulmonic valve – located between the right ventricle and the pulmonary trunk.

b.) Aortic valve - located between the left ventricle and aorta

Murmurs are caused by diseases of the valves or other structural abnormalities. The heart sounds are produced by the closure of the valves:

S1 – first heart sound is due to the closure of the mitral and tricuspid valves.

S2 – second heart sound is due to the closure of the aortic and pulmonic valves.

The vena cavae are two major blood vessels that collect deoxygenated blood. They are referred to as the superior vena cava and the inferior vena cava. The latter receives deoxygenated blood from the lower body parts of the body while the former receives blood from the upper extremities, neck and head.

2. Coronary Circulation

Coronary circulation is the blood movement through the heart tissues. Goldberger (2012, p. 17) states that coronary circulation can also be seen as blood circulation within the blood vessels of the myocardium (muscles of the heart). The coronary arteries are blood vessels that enrich the myocardium with oxygen and nutrients, while the coronary veins are blood vessels that remove deoxygenated blood from the heart. Epicardial coronary arteries are found on the surface of the heart and regulate the levels of coronary blood flow to the appropriate levels as required by the heart.

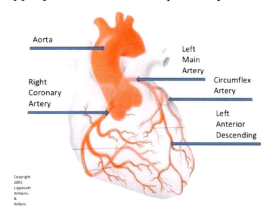

Sub-endocardial coronary arteries run inside myocardium. Coronary arteries are the only arteries that supply blood to the myocardium. They are seen as end circulation which means that blood supply redundancy is very little; hence, blocked vessels could be grave. Coronary arteries are characteristically narrow.

The right and left coronary arteries of the heart branch from the aorta emanating from aortic valve. The right coronary artery has several branches that supply the right ventricle with blood. The right coronary artery has branches known as posterior interventricular branches that nourish the left ventricle with blood. The left coronary artery supply blood to the left side of the heart and appears larger than the right coronary artery.

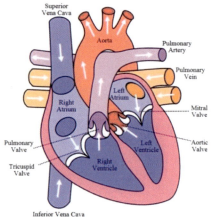

As a result, the left coronary artery require rigorous flow of blood. The left coronary artery branches into the circumflex and anterior interventricular arteries. The anterior interventricular artery supplies blood to ventricular septum and ventricles. The circumflex through left atrium and left ventricle nourish the left chambers and links with the posterior of the heart and the right coronary artery.

3. Heart Physiology

The heart being a muscular organ is always pumping blood to different parts of the body. The tissues that make up the cardiac muscles are strong and facilitate rhythmic contraction and relaxation movements the entire lifetime of a human being. The movements that describe the movements of the heart are systolic and diastolic.

Systole occurs when the heart contracts while diastole happens when the heart relaxes. The left ventricle forces blood into aorta at the same time that blood is forced from the right ventricle into pulmonary artery. When the ventricles contract, pressure increases. The pressure is referred to as systolic pressure.

Diastole causes relaxation of ventricular muscles. When the ventricles relax, the space for receiving blood from the two atria is created. Diastolic pressure is created because pressure decreases after the ventricles relax.

The muscle tissue of the heart has nerve fibers that make up a network. The network of nerves facilitates relaxation and contraction of the heart by enabling the cardiac muscles flow efficiently in a rhythmic manner. The coordination of the muscles causes the heart to have pumping strokes that appear wave-like. The heart septum which divides the heart does not allow the left and the right side of the heart to communicate directly. If there is a communication between the two sides, a septum defect could be the cause.

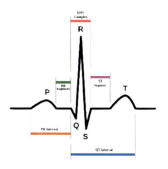

4. Basic Electrophysiology

Josephson (2001, p. 17) notes that, electrophysiology is a study of the human heart as it relates to the electrical conduction system of the heart. The primary characteristics of the cardiac cells are:

1. *Automaticity* – This is the ability of the cardiac pacemaker cells to spontaneously initiate their own electrical impulse without being stimulated from another source. Sites that possess this characteristic are the SA node, AV junction, and the Purkinje fibers.

2. *Excitability* – Also referred to as irritability. This characteristic is shared by all cardiac cells and it is the ability to respond to external stimulus: electrical, chemical, and mechanical.

3. *Conductivity* – This is the ability of all cardiac cells to receive an electrical stimulus and transmit the stimulus to the other cardiac cells.

4. *Contractility* -- This is the ability of the cardiac cells to shorten and cause cardiac muscle contraction in response to an electrical stimulus. This characteristic can be enhanced through administration of certain medications, such as digitalis, dopamine and epinephrine.

Conduction System of the Heart

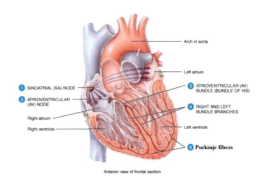

According to Baltazar (2009, p. 1), the heart consists of an electrical conduction system. The electrical conduction system consists of sinoatrial (SA) node, atrioventricular node, AV bundle, the bundle Branches (right and left), and purkinje fibres.

See this YouTube video

http://www.youtube.com/watch?v=te_SY3MeWys

SA Node

Found in the upper posterior portion of the right atrial wall just below the opening of the superior vena cava. It is the primary pacemaker of the heart and has a normal firing rate of 60-100 beats per minute.

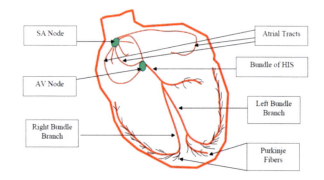

Internodal pathways

Consists of anterior, middle and posterior divisions that distribute electrical impulse generated by the SA node throughout the right and left atria to the atrioventricular (AV) node.

AV Junction:
AV node

Located at the posterior septal wall of the right atrium just above the tricuspid valve.

There is a 1/10th of a second delay of electrical activity at this level to allow blood to flow from the atria to the ventricles.

Bundle of His

Found at the superior portion of the interventricular septum, it is the pathway that leads out

of the SA node. It has an ability to initiate electrical impulses with an intrinsic firing rate of 40-60 beats per minute.

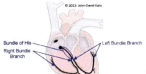

Bundle branches

Located at the interventricular septum, the bundle of His divides into the right and left bundle branches, the function of which is to conduct the electrical impulse to the Purkinje fibers.

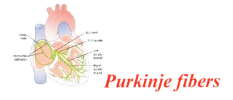

Purkinje fibers

Found within the ventricular endocardium, it consists of a network of small conduction fibers that delivers the electrical impulses to the ventricular myocardium. This network has the ability to initiate electrical impulses and act as a pacemaker if the higher-level pacemakers fail. The

intrinsic firing rate is 20-40 beats per minute.

Sinoatrial (SA) node sets the pace for the heart naturally, by releasing regular electrical impulses. It is located at the upper right section of the right atrium. Sinoatrial node initiates electrical impulse that causes every single heartbeat. The impulses are transmitted via the atria causing the contraction of the cardiac muscles in a rhythmic wave. The pace rate of the SA node are based on individual needs of the human body.

The impulse initiated by the sinoatrial node is received by the atrioventricular(AV) node. Atrioventricular(AV) node is located in the lower side and to the middle of the right atrium. The Atrioventricular node similarly transmits the impulse through the ventricular nerve network. The result is contractions by the ventricles that resemble waves. The network of electrical fibers or nerves in the ventricles exits the antrioventricular node either on the right or left bundle branches.

Simply said, there is something called the common bundle or atrioventricular bundle. The bundle branches into the right and left bundle branches with the left bundle going into the left ventricle and the right bundle going into the right ventricular. Impulse received through these nerve fibers result in the ventricular contractions.

Dubin (2000, p. 6) adds that, the heart being made up of up to a billion cells, consists of majority present in ventricular walls because of the amount of energy required to pump blood from the ventricles. Sinoatrial node rests when atrioventricular node is sending out impulse hence the heart does not stop for sinoatrial node to trigger another impulse. Therefore, there are two main stages: Depolarization(contraction) and Repolarization(Relaxation) of both the Atria and the ventricles.

Depolarization and Repolarization

Resting cardiac cells are negatively charged inside. When a cardiac

cell is stimulated, sodium ions rush into the cell and potassium leaks out, changing into positive the charge within. This electrical event is called depolarization and is expected to result in contraction. Depolarization flows from the endocardium to the myocardium to the epicardium.

During cell recovery, ions shift back to their original places and the cell recovers the negative charge inside. This is repolarization, and proceeds from the epicardium towards the endocardium. It results in myocardial relaxation.

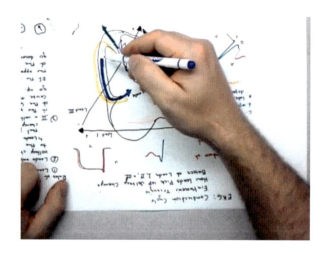

FUNDAMENTALS OF ELECTROCARDIOGRAM

Dubin (2000, p. 6) notes that, electrocardiogram is a machine that records information on the heart's electrical activity. Electrodes connecting the electrocardiogram machine and the patient's heart can provide a means of recording electrical activity for analysis. The EKG machine main objective is to detect the flow of the patient's heart electrical activity by measuring on the patient's skin.

The functions of an electrocardiogram include computing a person's heart rate on the monitor, the duration of depolarization, repolarization and the length of time it takes to conduct the impulses. The electrocardiogram assesses the pacemaker's motions and regularity. When the patient is being administered medications, the electrocardiogram can be used to evaluate the extent of response of the body or heart to the medication. An electrocardiogram machine can give baseline reading of the heart prior, during and following a treatment or medical procedure.

An EKG machine generates information useful for the cardiologist or physician that is specific and resourceful. The information may include details of the heart's orientation in the chest. Additionally, the effects of fluid and electrolyte imbalance can be detected on the EKG machine. Features such as damages of blood vessels or ischemic cardiac muscles can be viewed and the mass shown for easy assessment.

The electrocardiogram is limited and may not show enough data on myocardium. When conducting the procedure the blood pressure as well as pulse is evaluated to support evidence on mechanical activity of the heart.

THE ELECTROCARDIOGRAPHIC GRID AND WAVES

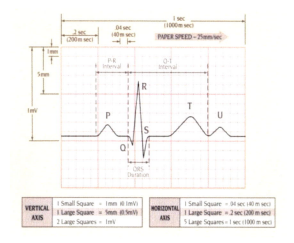

The electrocardiographic grid is a representation of measurement of voltage plotted on a vertical axis. The axis is on time. The voltage and time are detected when electrodes that are connected to the machine provide a difference. Usually, a distance is deflected depending on the voltage to be measured.

The electrocardiogram waves are recorded on a specified graph designed for recording the waves. The graph is constructed in a manner that grid like square boxes of one millimeter squared appear. The electrocardiogram machine records twenty five millimeters per second. Consequently, one millimeter on the horizontal is equal to 0.04 seconds to 0.2 seconds intervals. On the vertical grid the electrocardiogram takes the measurement of the height on the graph which is tantamount to 10 millimeter of the standard calibration.

Estimation of the rate can be achieved through a countdown using the grid. On the grid small and large boxes on the grid can be counted between the two P waves that follow and the two R waves that follow. For the small boxes the number between two following P waves for atrial together with the number of squares between of two following R waves for ventricles rates are used. There are other methods to determine the heart rate like the R-R interval, 60-seconds times 10 interval, etc.

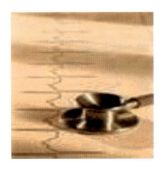

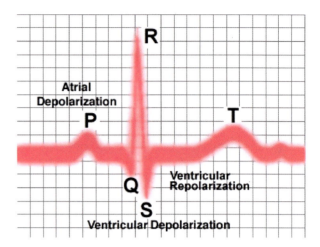

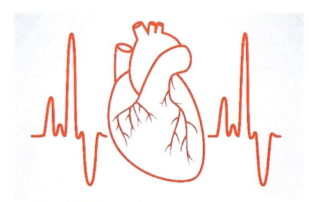

Definition of waves, segments, intervals and junctions

Waves in an electrocardiogram are in the form of P, T or QRS waves. P waves denote atria depolarization. QRS waves stand for ventricle depolarization and T represents repolarization of the ventricle. Atria repolarization is almost impossible to be detected or viewed and when detected it is denoted as T wave. There are other waves that can appear abnormally such as delta waves. Delta waves slight portion of the QRS wave. Epsilon wave is seen towards the end

72

of QRS wave. Osborn wave is also visible when QRS wave is ending in rigorous hypothermia (Canover 2003p. 41).

Wagner (2007, p. 11) notes that, a segment can be defined as the space between two waves. The PR segment begins after P wave and ends at the beginning of QRS complex. ST segments begin on end of QRS and ends at the beginning of T wave. In the cardiogram, a segment can also be described as isoelectric interval.

An interval can be defined as the region in a cardiogram that covers one segment with one or several waves. PR interval begins at beginning of the P wave and diminishes at the beginning of QRS. The difference between a PR interval and a PR segment is that a PR interval begins at the beginning of the P wave to the beginning of the Q wave, while a PR segment begins at the end of the P wave to the beginning of the Q wave. Some have questioned why it is not called the PQ interval, but NO, it is the PR interval. An interval can be interpreted as an impulse conducted from a section of atrium on the top towards the ventricle. QT interval begins where QRS starts and ends at the completion of T wave. An interval stands for the electrical systolic action performed by the heart. A junction is placed between a QRS and ST segment.

SIMPLY PUT:

Waveform: refers to movement away from the isoelectric line with either upward (positive) deflection or downward (negative) deflection.

Segment: line between two waveforms.

Interval: waveform plus a segment.

Complex: several waveforms

THE NORMAL ELECTROCARDIOGRAPH WAVES AND COMPLEXES

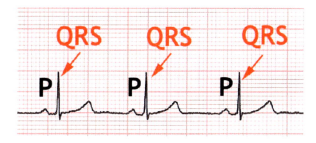

Normal electrocardiogram starts with a P wave that deflects atria depolarization (from right side to left then to inferiority) An active atrial depolarization appears on electrocardiogram as a P wave vertically in leads. The first precordial lead denoted as V1 is negative and signifies depolarization of posterity on the left side of the atrium. P wave amplitude does not exceed 2.5 millimeters and tenth of a second which is representative of a reduced amount of three boxes. Sometimes the P wave has a notch which separating left from right atrial actions. **P wave**: is the first deflection after the diastole, produced by atrial depolarization.

It is a smooth, round, not more than 2.5 mm high and no more than 0.11 sec

Positive in I,II, and V2 to V6. The normal P wave in standard, limb, and precordial leads does not exceed 0.11s in duration or 2.5mm in height. There is **no wave for atrial repolarization**, because is obscured by the larger QRS complex

PR segment detects isoelectric segment, which is deflected as well depolarized by abnormalities of atria caused by pericarditis or infarction of atrium. Normal PR measurements for the intervals are between 0.12 and 0.2 seconds.

QRS complexes timing is between 0.06 to 0.10 seconds. Q waves normally remains bellows 0.03 seconds and bellow 3milimetres depth. R wave remains within 20 to 25 millimeters height. QRS complex may be 30 to 105 degrees from the frontal axis indicating that there is a positive in the leads for the complexes. T wave faces identical direction with the QRS. The QT interval rate is subject to heart rate with the average normal heart beat being 70 beats per minute (Josephson, 2001, p. 57).

QRS complex Represents ventricular depolarization (activation). The ventricle is depolarized from the endocardium to the myocardium, to the epicardium. Normal duration is no more than 0.1 sec (otherwise stated as "less than .12 sec").

Q (q) wave: the initial negative deflection produced by ventricular depolarization.

R (r) wave: the first positive deflection produced by ventricular depolarization.

S (s) wave: the first negative deflection produced by the ventricular depolarization that follows the first positive deflection, (R) wave.

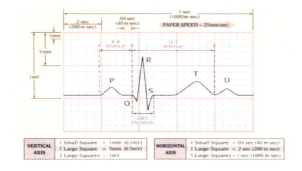

Ventricular Repolarization:

a. T wave: The first wave after the QRS complex has the following characteristics.

The deflection produced by ventricular repolarization. It is slightly asymmetric

No more than 5 mm in height.

b. U wave: Is the deflection seen following the T wave but preceding the diastole.

Represents repolarization of Purkinje fibers

Round and symmetric less than 1.5 mm in height. A prominent U wave is due to hypokalemia (low potassium, blood level).

THE NORMAL EKG SEGMENTS, INTERVALS AND JUNCTIONS

- **PR segment** this segment is measured from the end of the P wave to the beginning of the QRS complex. Represents depolarization of AV node and its delay and depolarization of the Bundle of His and the Bundle Branches.

- **ST segment** This segment represents the time of ventricular contraction and the beginning of repolarization of both ventricles. It is measured from end of QRS to the beginning of the T wave. The point where QRS complex and the ST segment meet is called "the junction" or "J point". ST segment is the most sensitive part of EKG changed by cardiac ischemia.

a. **PR Interval** Is defined as P wave plus PR segment and is measured from the beginning of P wave to the beginning of QRS complex. The normal interval is 0.12 – 0.2 sec.

b. **QT Interval** It represents the total ventricular activity (ventricular depolarization PLUS ventricular repolarization), and it is measured from the beginning of QRS to the end of T wave. The normal duration of this interval depends on the age and the HR.

c. **RR Interval.** It is important to determine the HR and its regularity.

RR interval: this is the interval between two R waves.

d. **J (RST) junction:** point at which QRS complex ends and ST segment begins.

e. **ST segment:** from J point to the onset of the T wave. This segment is compared to the PR segment to help identify myocardial ischemia or injury.

ANALYZING THE EKG STRIP

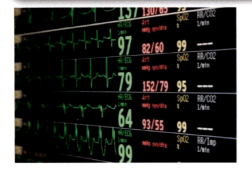

There are five steps that can be used for strip interpretation. The kind of rhythm determines the course of treatment to be administered. In the first stage, the electrocardiogram technician checks the rhythm to asses if the rhythm is normal or irregular. They assess if the rate is very fast, medium speed or too slow. 60 to 100 beats are considered the most appropriate hemodynamic hemorrhage. When the rate is below 60 beats or exceeds 100 beats, hemodynamic instability can be experienced.

The second stage is to evaluate if the heart rhythm is regular. The rhythms emanate from pace setters and are transmitted regularly. Irregular rhythm suggests that the beats are not released regularly and there could be abnormal beats which could be caused by certain conditions.

The third step involves examining all the components and the shape of waveforms. Check the measurement of the waves against the normal values like shape and duration.

The fourth step involves checking the position of the P wave. The electrocardiogram technologist finds out if P wave are present before the QRS complex, which denotes normal function of conduction from atria to ventricle. When p wave does not appear, the impulse could be emanating from a different part of the heart.

The final step establishes if all the complexes are alike. In a normal conduction each beat follow a similar pattern. Complexes that are diverse could indicate that impulses could be passing in wrong pathways.

Simply put:

1. **6 second Method**: The number of QRS complexes between 6 sec marks on the EKG paper is multiplied by 10. Used generally for estimating slow or irregular rhythms.

2. **Large Boxes Method**: count the number of large boxes between two consecutive RR (one RR interval) and divide into 300 for the ventricular rate; and count large boxes between two consecutive P waves for the atrial rate. Used mainly in regular rhythms.

3. **Small Boxes**: One minute has 1500 small boxes (0.04 sec). Count the number of small boxes between an RR interval and divide into 1500. This method is more accurate and is used for *regular rhythms only.*

4. **Sequence Method**: Select the R that falls on a dark vertical line. Number the next consecutive dark line as 300, 150, 100, 75, 60, and 50. Note where the next R wave falls in relation to the dark lines. That is the heart rate.

B. Assess Rhythm/ Regularity

The HR is considered regular if all the RR or PP intervals on the EKG leads are equal. If there are changes in their durations the rhythm is irregular.

C. Identify and examine the P waves:

Identify the P waves, PP interval and measure the size of the P wave in different leads.

D. Assess intervals (PR, QRS, QT):

Measure each of these intervals and determine if they are normal.

E. Evaluate ST segments and T waves.

ST segment elevation or depression and/or T wave abnormalities can suggest the presence of myocardial ischemia or injury.

F. General Evaluation and Conclusion:

Notify the doctor for any abnormality that you can find on the EKG strip.

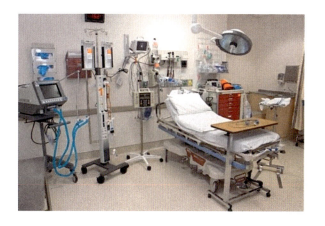

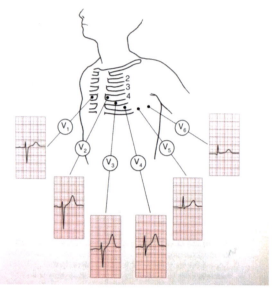

EKG Interpretation and Pathology Recordings

Cardiac arrhythmias are due to the following mechanisms:

Arrhythmias of sinus origin - where electrical flow follows the usual conduction pathway but is too fast, too slow, or irregular. Normal sinus rate is 60-100 beats per minute. If the rate goes beyond 100 per minute, it is called sinus tachycardia. If the rate goes below 60 per minute, it is referred to as sinus bradycardia.

Ectopic rhythms - electrical impulses originate from somewhere else other than the sinus node.

Conduction blocks - electrical impulses go down the usual pathway but encounter blocks and delays.

Pre-excitation syndromes - the electrical impulses bypass the normal pathway and, instead, go down an accessory shortcut.

Randal (2004, p. 54) mentions that when interpreting electrocardiogram, it is important to identify the normal behavior of the heart, that is the baseline method. A heart in good condition will have a Normal Sinus Rhythm. Any deviation from a normal sinus rhythm is usually a thing of concern. Some deviations like sinus dysrhythmia are of low concern while rhythms like Ventricular fibrillation are life threatening emergencies. Let us take a look at some common EKG Strips.

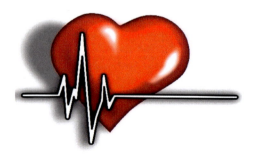

Normal Sinus Rhythm

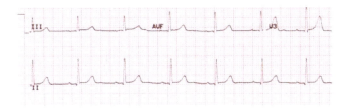

Originated from the SA Node and has the following characteristics:

a. Heart Rate of 60 – 100 bpm

b. Similar P waves in all the leads in front of all QRS complexes

c. A constant PR interval of 0.12 to 0.2 sec in all the leads,

d. Regular rhythm

e. QRS complex < 0.12

f. QT interval < 0.40

Sinus Bradycardia

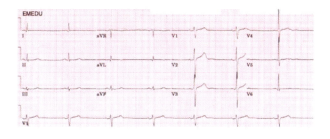

Bradycardia may be normal for athletes. It may also be normal in some individuals during sleep. Causes include vomiting, bearing down to have a bowel movement or diseases like myocardial infarction, obstructive jaundice and increased intracranial pressure. Medications such as digitalis, calcium-channel blockers and other anti-arrhythmic medications can also contribute to this rhythm. Features include:

a. HR less than 60 bpm

b. Normal equal P and QRS in all the leads, as well as normal PR intervals

c. . Bradycardia decreases the blood flow in the brain and other body tissues.

One can say that Sinus Bradycardia has the features of Normal Sinus Rhythm except a heart rate lower than 60 beats per minutes.

Sinus Tachycardia

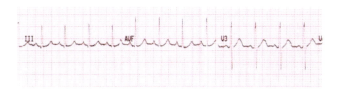

During stress and exercise, Sinus Tachycardia is normal. If Sinus Tachycardia persists at rest, conditions such as fever, dehydration, blood loss, anemia, anxiety, heart failure, hypermetabolic states and consumptions of stimulants such as cocaine, methamphetamine, etc may be the cause.

Drugs that can cause Sinus Tachycardia include: atropine, isoproterenol, epinephrine, dopamine, dobutamine, norepinephrine, nitroprusside and caffeine. Sinus Tach increases the heart's need for oxygen. Treatment includes finding out the underlying cause and treating it. Drugs of choice include: digitalis, beta-blockers, calcium-channel blockers, sedatives and other antiarrhythmic medications. Features include:

a. HR: 100 - 150 bpm

b. Normal equal P and QRS in all the leads, as well as normal PR intervals (0.12-0.20sec)

c. PR interval: 0.12-0.20 sec

d. QRS: < 0.12

Rhythm: Regular.

Sinus Tach originates from the SA Node.

Supraventricular Tachycardia (Life Threatening)

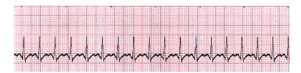

Atrial Tachycardia (AT) is caused by an irritable focus in the atria that fires electrical impulses after the normal firing of the SA node pacemaker. **HR is regular between 150 and 250 bpm.**

AV Reentry Tachycardia is caused when the electrical impulse passes through a passage other than AV node. Cardiac rhythm is regular but up to 250 bpm. P waves are often hidden by the QRS complexes or the QRS complexes that follow a P wave are different and with different PR interval (AV Nodal Reentry Tachycardia **AVNRT**).

In cases with **AV Reentry Tachycardia (AVRT) QRS** complexes are greater than 0.12 sec with a slurred up strike (delta wave) seen in one or more leads.

Atrial flutter

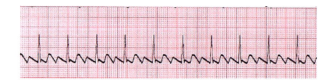

Atrial Flutter: Notice that there are no more "P" waves, instead a typical saw-tooth-like wave, called "F" wave is seen in the above recording. This rhythm leads to loss of atrial contraction resulting in decreased cardiac output 20-30%. Risks associated with this rhythm include: mural thrombi, hemodynamic instability, systemic or pulmonary embolism, etc. It is a life threatening situation. Cardioversion is usually done if it is an acute arrhythmia. If it is a chronic rhythm that is not responsive to medications, it is important that the patient be evaluated and possibly placed on an anticoagulant medication.

a. Atrial Flutter is characterized by rapid depolarization of a single atrial focus at a rate of 250-350 bpm.

b. Because the AV node cannot transmit every impulse at excessive rates, there is typically a slower ventricular rate (often appearing as a 2:1, 3:1, 4:1, etc. conduction ratio).

c. Typical **saw-toothed waves,** named "F" waves, followed by almost normal QRS complexes with a slower rate are seen in all the leads.

Atrial Fibrillation

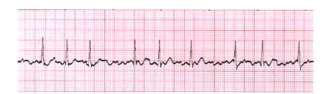

There are no "P" waves, instead they are substituted by small trembling waves, while QRST complex are almost normal and fired with a different rate.

Atrial fibrillation is caused by multiple irritable sites all over the atria firing at a rate exceeding 350 bpm. These rapid impulses cause quivering (fibrillation) of the muscular fibers, which results in a drastic decrease in the cardiac output, blood stagnation and the formation of a clot. Cardiac output is reduced with the loss of "Atrial Kick" because the atria are not contracting. If the ventricular rate are also fast, there will be further decreased cardiac output. The patient is at risk of pulmonary embolism or stroke. Causes: MI, Rheumatic Heart Disease, COPD, CHF, Ischemic Chest Trauma, CAD and open heart Surgery. Cardioversion is usually done in acute cases.

- No identifiable P waves can be seen, *fibrillatory erratic "f" waves* are seen in all the leads. Ventricular rhythm is very irregular, with a much slower rate than the atria. This is seen in all leads.

- Controlled atrial fibrillation: Average ventricular rate is less than 100 bpm.

- Uncontrolled atrial fibrillation: Average ventricular rate is over 100 bpm.

Premature Ventricular Complex

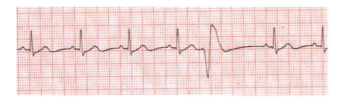

Notice the difference between the normal QRS complexes and the wide inverted abnormal QRS of the PVC and the full compensatory pause.

A premature ventricular complex arises from an irritable site within the ventricles. PVCs can appear as single, couplets, or triplets. Six or more PVCs occurring in a row are considered a run of V-Tach. PVC may appear in the same shape or in different shapes. When they appear in the same shape, they are believed to arise from a common point or focus, therefor are referred to as unifocal PVCs, but when they arise from different foci, they are referred to as multifocal PVCs.

The QRS of PVC is typically greater than 0.12 sec because the ventricular depolarization is abnormal or *aberrant*. The origin is usually ventricular/purkinje fibres. Causes: Increased catecholamines as seen in heightened emotions, stimulants such as coffee, nicotine, ethanol, cocaine, amphetamins, AMI, CHF, digitalis, increased vagal tones, hypoxia, acidosis, hypokalemia, hypomagnesemia, acidosis, ischemia, hypoxia and open heart surgery. T waves are usually in opposite direction of the QRS complex. A full compensatory pause usually follows a PVC. The rate and the PR interval are that of the underlying rhythm. The most important treatment is to find out and treat the underlying causes. Drugs of choice include beta blockers, procainamide, lidocaine, amiodarone, etc.

Ventricular Tachycardia

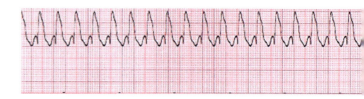

Ventricular Tachycardia (V-Tach) is characterized by 3 or more PVC's in a row at a rate over 100 bpm. If V-Tach occurs for more than 30 sec is called *sustained Ventricular Tachycardia.* The main characteristics of this rhythm are: Regular fast rhythm 100 to 250 bpm, No P waves or P waves may be present if SA node is functional, however, there is no relation to the QRS Wide, bizarre QRS complexes > 0.12 with T waves pointing in opposite direction from main QRS direction (T waves may be difficult to identify). If QRS complexes are different in size it is called *Polymorphic V-Tach* or "Torsades de Pointes".

Causes of V-Tach include hypoxia, acidosis, cardiomyopathy, mitral valve prolapse, digitalis toxicity, antiarrhythmics, electrolyte imbalance, liquid protein diets, increased intracranial pressure and central nervous system disorders. The longer a patient stays in V-Tach, the more difficult it is to convert to a normal rhythm. Stable patients may be medicated to attempt a chemical conversion. Unstable patients are treated promptly with defibrillation. **It is a life threatening emergency.**

Ventricular Fibrillation (Life threatening)

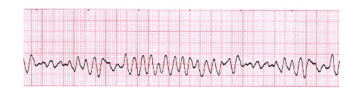

It is produced by multiple electrical sites firing electrical impulses at the same time resulting in quivering of the ventricles myocardial muscle fibers, but not a uniform contraction.

The rhythm is a chaotic deflection of different waves that vary in size, shape and duration. There are no normal visible waves. There is no contraction, there is no blood ejected in the blood vessels, so the blood can clot. This is a medical emergency, which requires defibrillation and CPR.

Asystole (No electrical activity in the heart)

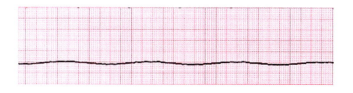

First Degree Heart Block, Type I

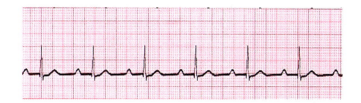

It is characterized by a delay of impulses at the level of AV node. . *PR interval is prolonged and is greater than 0.2 sec*

Second Degree Heart Block Type I

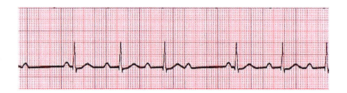

PR interval lengthens in each interval until one QRS disappears

Type II Second Degree AV Block (Mobitz II)

It is a more serious pathology.

Conducted P waves have a constant PR interval; but there are always non-conducted P waves between cardiac cycles, usually producing a "conduction ratio" between atria and ventricles (i.e. 2 P waves for each QRS, or 3 P waves for each QRS)

Third Degree AV Block. This type of AV block is also called a Complete Heart Block, or CHB, because impulses generated by the SA node are completely blocked before reaching the ventricular muscle fibers. The atria and ventricles beat independently from each other. Second degree blocks can progress in third degree blocks, especially after an inferior MI (myocardial Infarction). The third degree block's characteristics are:

- ❖ Atrial rate is greater than ventricular rate
- ❖ P waves are normal, there are no measurable PR intervals.
- ❖ The atrial rhythm (P waves) is regular; AND the ventricular rhythm is regular (QRS complexes).

There is no relationship between P waves and QRS complexes. If the escape rhythm is junctional, the QRS complexes may appear normal in width and the ventricular rate may be slightly higher

If the escape rhythm is ventricular, the QRS complexes will be abnormally wide with a slower ventricular rate.

ARTIFACTS OF EKG RECORDING

SOMATIC TREMOR

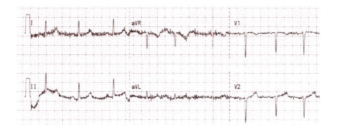

Wandering Baseline

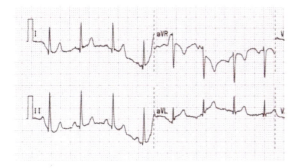

60 Cycle Circumference

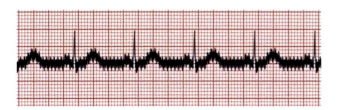

EKG AMBULATORY SYSTEMS:

The following are the basic requirements for ambulatory systems. They include consumption of power that is low, detection for low voltage power battery, ability to obtain the electrocardiogram leads simultaneously. Wireless communication, small in size, operation time of the battery should be a minimum of 24 hours continuously and obtain a recording ability with functions of display and enough storage in real time.

It consists of two blocks which are fitted with a transmitter and a receiver. The transmitters function is to condition, process, digitalize, encode and transmit to the electrocardiogram leads together with battery information to be received. The receiver detects information transmitted via the electrocardiogram where it is decoded. The Signal is send computer for recording display and storage.

CONCLUSION

An electrocardiogram technologist assists in the use of electrocardiogram machine in a physician's room or laboratory to generate information used for diagnosis. The human heart is made up of muscle tissue, located between the lungs and pump blood to different parts of the body. The electrocardiogram records hearts activity and presents them on a screen or recorded tape where the information is analyzed. The electrocardiogram records heart orientation, heart disturbance, effects of medication on heart and base line reading of heart activity. The electrocardiogram requires interpretation from an expert. Some abnormalities detected can be treated for patients to recover.

REFERENCES

Baltazar, R. F. (2009). *Basic and Bedside Electrocardiography*. New York: Lippincott Williams & Wilkins.

Canover, M. B. (2003) *Understanding Electrocardiography*. Philadelphia, PA: Mosby.

Dubin, D. (2000). *Rapid Interpretation of EKG's*. Florida, USA: Cover Publishing Company.

Ecman, M. (1990). *ECG interpretation*. New York: Springhouse Corporation.

Gomella, L. (2006). *Clinician's Pocket Reference*. New York: McGraw-Hill Medical.

Goldberger, A. L. (2012). *Clinical Electrocardiography: A Simplified Approach*. Philadelphia, PA: Saunders.

Hummel, J. D., Kalbfleisch, S. J. and J. M. Dillon. (1999). *Pocket Guide for Cardiac Electrophysiology*. Philadelphia: W. B. Saunders Company.

Josephson, M. E. (2001). *Clinical Cardiac Electrophysiology: Techniques and Interpretations*. Philadelphia: Lippincott Williams & Wilkins Publishers.

Randal, D. C. (2004). *ECG Interpretation*. Hayes Barton Press.

Wagner, G. S. (2007). *Marriott's Practical Electrocardiography*. New York: Lippincott Williams & Wilkins.

Section One Questions

1. Which of the following is an example of the duties of a Patient Care Technician?
   a. Handling basic paperwork
   b. Taking the vital signs of the patients
   c. Answering the phone
   d. All of the above are functions of a PCT

2. What is a thermometer used for?
   a. Assessing the pulse of a patient
   b. Measuring blood pressure of a patient
   c. Measuring body temperature
   d. Assessing the responsiveness of a patient

3. An oral thermometer produces a reading of 101 degrees Fahrenheit. This patient is:
   a. Febrile
   b. Afebrile
   c. Normal
   d. None of the above

4. A fever that remains constant is:
   a. Remittent
   b. Afebrile
   c. Continuous
   d. Intermittent

5. Who should have their temperatures taken orally?
   a. Elderly patients
   b. Patients receiving oxygen
   c. Teenage patients
   d. Patients with broken ribs

6. Which patients should not have temperatures taken rectally?
   a. Patients with NG tubes
   b. Patients with diarrhea
   c. Infants
   d. Patients who smoke

7. How should a pulse be taken?
   a. With the first two or three fingers for about thirty seconds
   b. With the third and fourth finger on the femoral artery
   c. With the thumb on the jugular
   d. With the thumb on the brachial artery

8. Which of the following counts as a respiration?
   a. An inhale
   b. An inhale and an exhale
   c. An exhale
   d. A cough

9. The apical pulse is taken:
   a. With the first and second finger
   b. Over the apex of the heart with the palm of the hand
   c. Over the apex of the heart with a stethoscope
   d. None of the above

10. The apical pulse is especially useful in:
    a. Infants or small children
    b. In the elderly
    c. In patients with brittle bones
    d. In patients going into fibrillation

11. When taking a pulse you should feel:
    a. On the radial artery which is located on the same side as the patient's pinky
    b. On the brachial artery on the back side of the arm
    c. On the temporal artery located on the forehead
    d. On the radial artery located on the same side as the patient's thumb

12. Tachypnea is characterized by:
    a. A rate of breathing greater than 40 breaths per minute
    b. A rate of breathing less than 10 breaths per minute
    c. A rate of breathing greater than 100 breaths per minute
    d. A rate of breathing less than 5 breaths per minute

13. A patient has a fever that has been fluctuating all day. However, the fever never returns to a baseline or a normal temperature. This is considered:
    a. Continuous fever
    b. Intermittent fever
    c. Remittent fever
    d. Afebrile fever

14. Apnea occurs when:
    a. The patient permanently stops breathing
    b. The patient temporarily has complete absence of breath
    c. The patient is in hysteria
    d. The patient is breathing normally

15. Bradypnea:
    a. Occurs when a patient hyperventilates
    b. Has a breathing rate of greater than 40 breaths per minute
    c. Is normal during a sleeping state
    d. Is never normal

16. Depth of respiration refers to:
    a. Number of breaths per minutes
    b. Amount of air inspired and expired
    c. Number of heartbeats per minute
    d. Amount of blood pumped through the heart per minute

17. Hypoventilation refers to a time when:
    a. Reduced air enters the lungs
    b. Increased air enters the lungs
    c. Normal amounts of air enters the lungs

    d. No air enters the lungs

18. Hypoventilation results in:
    a. Excess oxygen in the blood and decreased carbon dioxide in the blood
    b. Excess nitrogen in the blood and decreased carbon dioxide
    c. Decreased nitrogen in the blood and increased oxygen in the blood
    d. Decreased oxygen in the blood and increased carbon dioxide

19. Blood pressure can be described as:
    a. The distance pressurized blood will travel
    b. The amount of stress that veins can safely handle
    c. The amount of force exerted by blood on peripheral arteries
    d. None of the above

20. An instrument that measures blood pressure is known as a:
    a. Hypometer
    b. Sphygmomanometer
    c. Barometer
    d. Mercometer

21. Which artery does the blood pressure cuff center over?
    a. Jugular artery
    b. Femoral artery
    c. Antecubital artery
    d. Brachial artery

22. Failure to properly place the cuff can lead to:
    a. False diagnosis of high or low blood pressure
    b. Rupture of the veins
    c. Accurate diagnosis of high or low blood pressure
    d. Discomfort

23. Cuffs that are too small or narrow can lead to:
    a. Unusually low blood pressure readings
    b. Abnormal heart rate readings
    c. Unusually high blood pressure readings
    d. All of the above

24. Anthropometric measurements refers to:
    a. Measurements of the heart and lungs
    b. Comparative measurements of the body
    c. Comparative measurements of lung function
    d. All of the above

25. During the examination, the medical assistant will be responsible for:
    a. Room and patient preparation
    b. Patient examination
    c. Patient treatment
    d. Room maintenance

26. Which of the following does the physician use to make a diagnosis?

a. Patient history
b. Lab tests
c. Physical examination
d. All of the above

27. How would someone examine a patient using palpation?
    a. Listening to breath sounds
    b. Tapping on a patient's chest to listen to the sounds
    c. Feeling a pulse
    d. All of the above

28. Which position is the most commonly used for patient examination?
    a. The vertical recumbent position
    b. The horizontal flat dorsal position
    c. Vertical pineal dorsal position
    d. The horizontal recumbent position

29. Which of the following is used for pelvic exams?
    a. Dorsal lithotomy position
    b. The horizontal recumbent position
    c. The vertical recumbent position
    d. Dilliad's position

30. A patient comes in for an exam. The patient is having trouble breathing. Which position do you place the patient in?
    a. Vertical recumbent position
    b. Fowler's position
    c. Dilliard's position
    d. Any of the above

31. Which position is used for a rectal exam?
    a. Fowler's position
    b. Prone position
    c. Sim's position
    d. Dilliard's position

32. Most accidents occur because:
    a. The patient does not cooperate
    b. Rules are overlooked or ignored
    c. Healthcare professionals don't care
    d. None of the above

33. Which of the following is an example of a hazard in the healthcare setting?
    a. Electrical hazards
    b. Biological hazards
    c. Chemical hazards
    d. All of the above

34. A coworker has noticed a stripped cord connected to a bed. This is an example of:
    a. Electrical hazards
    b. Biological hazards
    c. Chemical hazards
    d. Neurological hazards

35. Someone has left out some strong cleaning supplies. This is an example of:
    a. Electrical hazards
    b. Biological hazards
    c. Chemical hazards

d. Neurological hazards

36. Someone has left out an uncapped, used sharp. This is an example of:
    a. Electrical hazards
    b. Biological hazards
    c. Chemical hazards
    d. Neurological hazards

37. A coworker has cut himself badly on a jagged piece of metal. You should:
    a. Have the coworker lie down
    b. Pour disinfectant on the wound
    c. Apply pressure and elevate the wound
    d. Perform CPR

38. A patient is on the floor with cold/clammy skin, blank expression, and shallow breathing. This patient possibly is suffering from:
    a. Shock
    b. Stroke
    c. Heart attack
    d. Sun poisoning

39. CPR stands for:
    a. Cardio-Palpitative Resuscitation
    b. Carotid-Pulmonary Recognizance
    c. Cardio-Pulmonary Resuscitation
    d. Carotid-Palliative Recognizance

40. An influenza virus is an example of:
    a. An agent
    b. A portal of exit
    c. A mode of transmission
    d. A portal of entry

41. Which of the following is not an example of a portal of entry?
    a. A scratch on the hand
    b. Intact skin
    c. A mucous membrane
    d. Respiratory tract

42. Which of the following is not an example of a mode of transmission?
    a. Wearing gloves
    b. Being sneezed on
    c. Contact with blood
    d. Touching an infected surface

43. Which of the following means "the destruction of pathogenic microorganisms after they leave the body"?
    a. Vector transmission
    b. Asymmetry
    c. Medical Asepsis
    d. Organ Sepsis

44. When disinfecting items you should:
    a. Use chemicals on every item to be disinfected
    b. Put everything into a cleaning oven
    c. Wipe everything down with water
    d. Use chemicals only on inanimate objects

45. Which item would not be eligible to be cleaned with boiling water?
    a. An oral thermometer

b. A pair of utility scissors
c. A reflex hammer
d. A mug

46. Surgical instruments are placed in an autoclave. This is an example of:
    a. Dry heat sterilization
    b. Chemical sterilization
    c. Steam sterilization
    d. Gas sterilization

47. A wheelchair is placed in a chamber for sterilization. This is most likely an example of:
    a. Dry heat sterilization
    b. Chemical sterilization
    c. Steam sterilization
    d. Gas sterilization

48. The most important way of fighting infection is:
    a. Dry heat sterilization
    b. Hand washing
    c. Cleaning things with bleach
    d. All of the above

49. You must wear a face shield for performing a procedure. This is an example of:
    a. Isolation
    b. Medical asepsis
    c. Barrier protection
    d. Contact asepsis

50. Standard precautions include which of the following?
    a. Wearing gloves
    b. Wearing face shields when necessary
    c. Disposing of sharps without recapping
    d. All of the above

51. In order to prevent airborne diseases from spreading you should use:
    a. Universal precautions
    b. Contact precautions
    c. Airborne precautions
    d. All of the above

52. You catch a cold after you drink after your daughter. This is an example of:
    a. Airborne contamination
    b. Indirect contact transmission
    c. Direct contact transmission
    d. Vector transmission

53. A patient contracted a disease from the hospital. This is an example of:
    a. A nosocomial infection
    b. Direct contact transmission
    c. Barrier protection
    d. A susceptible host

54. A child develops a rash after playing closely with another child. This could be an example of:
    a. Direct contact transmission
    b. Airborne transmission
    c. Vector transmission
    d. Indirect contact transmission

55. A virus is an example of a:
    a. Susceptible host
    b. An agent
    c. A vector
    d. Portal of exit

56. Standard precautions are aimed at:
    a. Preventing the spread of infectious agents as they exit the reservoir
    b. Preventing the spread of infectious as they enter the susceptible host
    c. Preventing the spread of infectious agents as they travel through the air
    d. None of the above

57. When a person appears to be in shock you should:
    a. Have the person sit up and elevate the arms
    b. Have the person stand up and elevate the arms
    c. Have the person lay down and elevate the feet
    d. None of the above

58. When should you wash your hands?
    a. Before and after speaking with the patient
    b. Before and after entering a room
    c. After eating and using the bathroom
    d. After leaving the hospital

59. To avoid chemical hazards you should always:
    a. Store chemicals with non-hazardous materials
    b. Pour chemicals into clear bottles
    c. Label all chemicals with the MSDS
    d. All of the above

60. In order to avoid biological hazards you should:
    a. Incinerate any non-cleanable materials
    b. Sterilize any materials that can be sterilized
    c. Wash hands before and after each procedure
    d. All of the above

61. To avoid electrical hazards you should:
    a. Never use extension cords
    b. Replace any cords that are bare or have the wire showing
    c. Unplug electrical equipment before servicing
    d. All of the above

62. When an accident occurs you should:
    a. Attempt to clean up the mess before anyone notices
    b. Talk about it with a co-worker
    c. Report it to a supervisor
    d. Leave it for someone else

63. A patient needs to be examined in the posterior aspect. Which position should you use for this patient?
    a. Trendelenburg
    b. Prone position
    c. Sim's position

d. None of the above

64. Which of the following would a medical assistant do for the patient?
    a. Collect vitals
    b. Explain the procedure
    c. Positioning and draping the patient
    d. All of the above

65. Which of the following is not an anthropometric measurement?
    a. Lucidity
    b. Weight
    c. Height
    d. Head circumference

66. How fast should a blood pressure cuff deflate?
    a. 1-2 mmHg per second
    b. 2-3 mmHg per second
    c. 4-5 mmHg per second
    d. 6-7 mmHg per second

67. A state where increased air is entering the lungs is called:
    a. Hypopnea
    b. Hyperpnoea
    c. Hyperventilation
    d. Hypoventilation

68. Cheyne-Stokes refers to:
    a. Regular pattern of irregular breathing
    b. Irregular pattern of regular breathing
    c. Regular pattern of regular breathing
    d. Irregular pattern of irregular breathing

69. Orthopnea refers to:
    a. Trouble breathing because of problems with the rib bones
    b. Regular breathing in an inverted position
    c. Difficulty breathing when not upright
    d. Difficulty breathing when upright

70. Apnea refers to:
    a. A period of increased breathing, then returning to normal
    b. A period if no breath
    c. A period if decreased breath depth
    d. None of the above

71. When using a rectal thermometer:
    a. All patients are eligible for rectal thermometers
    b. Only babies should have rectal temperatures taken
    c. Only elderly patients should have rectal temperatures taken
    d. Patients with heart disease should not have rectal temperatures taken

72. If a patient has just been drinking or smoking you should:
    a. Take temperature orally anyway
    b. Wait thirty minutes and then take his/her temperature
    c. Wait ten minutes and then take temperature rectally

d. None of the above

73. A patient is described as afebrile. This patient is:
    a. Having heart trouble
    b. Having breathing trouble
    c. Has a normal body temperature
    d. Has fertility problems

74. A patient has an axillary temperature of 98 degrees Fahrenheit. This patient:
    a. Has a normal body temperature
    b. Has a low body temperature
    c. Has a high body temperature
    d. Should be tested with an oral thermometer

75. Which of the following is not a place to take a temperature?
    a. Axillary area
    b. Rectal area
    c. Antecubital area
    d. Ear

76. Social history includes:
    a. Summary of family health problems
    b. Lifestyle
    c. Past surgeries
    d. Chief complaint

77. Medical history includes:
    a. Past surgeries
    b. Major illnesses
    c. Medications
    d. All of the above

78. Family history includes:
    a. Health problems of parents
    b. Past surgeries
    c. Lifestyle
    d. Major illnesses

79. A systematic check of each organ and system along with documenting positive and negative results is called a:
    a. Review of the body
    b. Review of systems
    c. Review of the patient
    d. None of the above

80. A Medical Assistant might:
    a. Collect specimens
    b. Instruct a patient about medications
    c. Gather vitals
    d. All of the above

81. Medical assistants do not:
    a. Make a diagnosis
    b. Assist the physician
    c. Dispose of contaminated supplies
    d. Prepare patients for XRays

82. Medical assistants might:
    a. Do medical transcription
    b. Maintain medical records
    c. Manage finances
    d. All of the above

83. An explanation of the chief complaint along with the symptoms and duration is part of:
    a. Social history
    b. Family history

c. History of present illness
d. Medical history

84. Which of the following is not a vital sign?
    a. Respiration
    b. Weight
    c. Pulse
    d. Temperature

85. Which of the following is the least accurate way to attain a temperature?
    a. Rectally
    b. Orally
    c. Ear
    d. Axillary

86. The normal pulse ranges between:
    a. 20 and 40 BPM
    b. 30 and 70 BPM
    c. 60 and 100 BPM
    d. 90 and 130 BPM

87. When taking a blood pressure with a stethoscope and a sphygmomanometer:
    a. Note the level at which two consecutive beats occur and the level at which all sounds disappear
    b. Note the level at which the blood pressure cuff becomes too tight
    c. Note the level at which the cuff completely deflates
    d. None of the above

88. To avoid biological hazards you should:
    a. Always wear gloves
    b. Disinfect the work area
    c. Wash hands
    d. All of the above

89. A person sneezes and germs are spread through drops across the room. This is an example of:
    a. Airborne transmission
    b. Droplet transmission
    c. Contact transmission
    d. All of the above

90. A person is blankly staring, has a rapid and weak pulse, and increased, shallow breathing. This person may be suffering from:
    a. Cheyne-Stokes
    b. Shock
    c. Stroke
    d. Hematoma

91. If it is necessary to use a bleach solution for disinfecting it should be diluted:
    a. 1 bleach : 1 water
    b. 2 bleach : 1 water
    c. 4 bleach : 1 water
    d. 1 bleach : 10 water

92. Airborne precautions are used to isolate:
    a. All patients that might have any contagion
    b. Any patients that might pose a direct contact threat
    c. Any patient that might offer

airborne infection
d. Only young and elderly patients

93. Contact precautions are used when:
a. The patient might have a disease that is spread through direct contact
b. A patient might have an airborne disease
c. A patient might have a droplet disease
d. None of the above

94. Standard precautions are:
a. Precautions used only for contagious patients
b. Precautions used only when the caregiver is ill
c. Precautions used on all patients
d. Precautions used only on foreign patients

95. Which of the following is the most important and most basic way of preventing disease transmission?
a. Face masks
b. Gloves
c. Face shields
d. Hand washing

96. Dry heat sterilization would be used for:
a. Cleaning hands
b. Cleaning wheelchairs
c. Cleaning instruments that easily corrode
d. Cleaning beds

97. A fungi is an example of a:
a. Vector
b. Agent
c. Reservoir
d. Host

98. A person is bleeding. This is an example of:
a. Susceptible host
b. Shock
c. External hemorrhaging
d. All of the above

99. When should you wash your hands?
a. Before and after speaking with the patient
b. Before and after entering a room
c. After eating and using the bathroom
d. After leaving the hospital

100. Which of the following pressurizes steam in order to sterilize?
a. Chemical sterilization
b. Dry heat sterilization
c. Steam sterilization
d. Water sterilization

Section One Answers

1. D
2. C
3. A
4. C
5. B
6. B
7. A
8. B
9. C

#	Ans	#	Ans
10.	A	47.	D
11.	D	48.	B
12.	A	49.	C
13.	C	50.	D
14.	B	51.	C
15.	C	52.	B
16.	B	53.	A
17.	A	54.	A
18.	D	55.	B
19.	C	56.	A
20.	B	57.	C
21.	D	58.	B
22.	A	59.	C
23.	C	60.	D
24.	B	61.	D
25.	A	62.	C
26.	D	63.	B
27.	B	64.	D
28.	D	65.	A
29.	A	66.	B
30.	B	67.	C
31.	C	68.	A
32.	B	69.	C
33.	D	70.	B
34.	A	71.	D
35.	C	72.	B
36.	B	73.	C
37.	C	74.	A
38.	A	75.	C
39.	C	76.	B
40.	A	77.	D
41.	B	78.	A
42.	A	79.	B
43.	C	80.	D
44.	D	81.	A
45.	A	82.	D
46.	C	83.	C

84. B
85. D
86. C
87. A
88. D
89. B
90. B
91. D
92. C
93. A
94. C
95. D
96. C
97. B
98. C
99. B
100. C

Questions for Section two

1. Which of the following machines detects the heart's electrical signals?
    a. The defibrillator
    b. The EKG
    c. The CT
    d. The respirator

2. Which of the following are responsibilities of the EKG technician?
    a. Moving patients
    b. Making patients comfortable
    c. Attaching electrodes
    d. All of the above

3. Which test is performed while the patient is on a treadmill in order to provide readings at diversified physical force?
    a. The CT test
    b. The Physical
    c. The Stress test
    d. The Psychological test

4. Which test monitor's the patient's heart readings for an entire day?
    a. Stress test
    b. Holter monitor
    c. EKG
    d. Cardiological movement test

5. The innermost layer of the heart is the:
    a. Epicardium
    b. Myocardium
    c. Endocardium
    d. None of the above

6. Fibrous pericardium helps the heart:
    a. Pump regularly
    b. Stay anchored to body parts
    c. Remain smooth
    d. None of the above

7. Pericardial fluid is located:
    a. Inside the ventrical
    b. Inside the atrium

c. Between the myocardium and endocardium
   d. Between fibrous and serous pericardium

8. Which portion of the heart receives deoxygenated blood?
   a. The right ventrical
   b. The left atrium
   c. The left ventrical
   d. The right atium

9. Which veins carry oxygenated blood?
   a. Jugular veins
   b. Pulmonary veins
   c. Coronary veins
   d. Vessical veins

10. Where is the tricuspid valve located?
    a. Between the right and left atrium
    b. Between the aorta and the heart
    c. Between the right atrium and the right ventricle
    d. Between the left atrium and the left ventricle

11. Diseases of valves are called:
    a. Hums
    b. Murmurs
    c. Skips
    d. Beats

12. Heart sounds are produced by:
    a. Valve closure
    b. Muscle contraction
    c. Muscle expansion
    d. Valve opening

13. The pulmonic valve is located:
    a. Between the aorta and the ventricles
    b. Between the right ventricle and the pulmonary trunk
    c. Between the left ventricle and the aorta
    d. Between the aorta and the pulmonary trunk

14. The aortic valve is located:
    a. Between the aorta and the vena cava
    b. Between the right ventricle and pulmonary trunk
    c. Between the left ventricle and aorta
    d. Between the aorta and the pulmonary trunk

15. Which node is the primary pacemaker of the heart?
    a. The ventricular node
    b. The atrial node
    c. The jugular node
    d. The sinoatrial node

16. What delivers electrical impulses to the ventricular myocardium through a network of fibers?
    a. Bundle branches
    b. Endothelial cells
    c. Purkinje fibers
    d. Endometrial fibers

17. Contractility refers to:
    a. The irritability of the cells
    b. The ability of the cells to communicate

c. The ability of the cells to expand and contract
d. The ability of the cells to conduct electrical impulses

18. Conductivity refers to:
    a. Irritability of the cells
    b. The ability of the cells to communicate
    c. The ability of the cells to expand and contract
    d. Ability of the cells to conduct electrical impulses

19. Which of the following statements is true?
    a. The SA node and the AV node fire simultaneously
    b. The SA node and the AV node control the heart valves
    c. The SA node and the AV node fire alternately of each other
    d. The SA node and the AV node control the vena cava

20. Which arteries are the only arteries to supply blood to the endocardium?
    a. Vena cava arteries
    b. Coronary arteries
    c. Jugular arteries
    d. Aorta

21. Systole occurs when:
    a. The heart contracts
    b. The heart relaxes
    c. The heart completes one contracting/relaxing cycle
    d. Blood moves through the veins

22. Diastole occurs when:
    a. The heart contracts
    b. The heart relaxes
    c. The heart skips a beat
    d. Blood moves through the arteries

23. Internodal pathways refers to:
    a. The electrical pathways from the brain to the heart
    b. The electrical pathways that send signals from the AV node to the SA node
    c. The electrical pathways that send signals from the SA node to the AV node
    d. The electrical pathways that move blood within the heart

24. What is located at the posterior septal wall of the right atrium just above the tricuspid valve?
    a. The SA node
    b. The AV node
    c. The Purkinje fibers
    d. The bundle of HIS

25. The electrical network within the heart:
    a. Spreads out through the heart in a web
    b. Runs in a straight line from top to bottom
    c. Runs in a circle around the heart
    d. Is one single point on the heart

26. Which node regulates heartrate?
    a. AV node
    b. Purkinje fibers
    c. SM node

d. SA node

27. Electrical impulses travel through the heart because of:
    a. Muscle contractions
    b. Depolarization and Repolarization
    c. Blood movement
    d. Oxygen in the blood

28. EKG's measure:
    a. The length of time it takes to depolarize and repolarize
    b. The duration of the impulses
    c. The length of time it takes to conduct impulses
    d. All of the above

29. The horizontal portion of the grid on an EKG represents:
    a. Time
    b. Heart size
    c. Electrical impulses
    d. Blood volume

30. P waves represent:
    a. Ventricle repolarization
    b. Ventricle depolarization
    c. Atrial depolarization
    d. Atrial repolarization

31. The QRS wave represents:
    a. Ventricle repolarization
    b. Ventricle depolarization
    c. Atrial depolarization
    d. Atrial repolarization

32. The T wave represents:
    a. Ventricle repolarization
    b. Ventricle depolarization
    c. Atrial depolarization
    d. Atrial repolarization

33. Which of the following cannot be viewed on an EKG?
    a. Ventricle repolarization
    b. Ventricle depolarization
    c. Atrial depolarization
    d. Atrial repolarization

34. A complex (ie a QRS complex) refers to:
    a. A line between waveforms
    b. A waveform plus a segment
    c. A single waveform
    d. Several waveforms

35. An interval on an EKG is:
    a. A line between waveforms
    b. A waveform plus a segment
    c. A single waveform
    d. Several waveforms

36. A segment on an EKG is:
    a. A line between waveforms
    b. A waveform plus a segment
    c. A single waveform
    d. Several waveforms

37. Why is there no wave for atrial repolarization?
    a. The atria don't repolarize
    b. The repolarization is obscured by the QRS
    c. The repolarization is obscured by the T wave

d. There is a wave for atrial repolarization if you look closely

38. The first step in analyzing an EKG is:
   a. Assess the rate
   b. Evaluate the heart rhythm
   c. Check the position of the P wave
   d. Check that all complexes are alike

39. The third step in analyzing an EKG is:
   a. Assess the rate
   b. Evaluate the heart rhythm
   c. Examine the components and shapes of the waveforms
   d. Check that all complexes are alike

40. When an electrical impulse originates from somewhere other than the SA node it is called:
   a. A normal sinus rhythm
   b. Ectopic rhythm
   c. Conduction block
   d. Pre-excitation syndrome

41. What is the name for a condition where electrical impulse travels down the normal pathways, but experience blocks or delays?
   a. A normal sinus rhythm
   b. Ectopic rhythm
   c. Conduction block
   d. Pre-excitation syndrome

42. What is it called when electrical impulses bypass the normal pathways and go down shortcuts?
   a. A normal sinus rhythm
   b. Ectopic rhythm
   c. Conduction block
   d. Pre-excitation syndrome

43. The following is an example of
   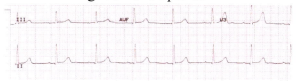
   a. Sinus bradycardia
   b. Sinus tachycardia
   c. Normal sinus rhythm
   d. Sinus arrhythmia

44. The following is an example of
   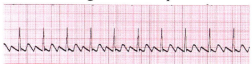
   a. Sinus bradycardia
   b. Atrial flutter
   c. Ventricular fibrillation
   d. Atrial fibrillation

45. The following is an example of
   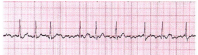
   a. Ventricular fibrillation
   b. Atrial fibrillation
   c. Atrial flutter
   d. Normal sinus rhythm

46. The following is an example of

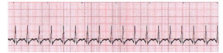

   a. Supraventricular tachycardia
   b. Atrial fibrillation
   c. Sinus tachycardia
   d. Atrial flutter

47. The following is an example of

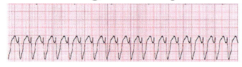

   a. Sinus tachycardia
   b. Atrial flutter
   c. Ventricular tachycardia
   d. Premature ventricular complex

48. The following is an example of

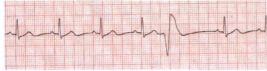

   a. Sinus tachycardia
   b. Atrial flutter
   c. Ventricular tachycardia
   d. Premature ventricular complex

49. The following is an example of

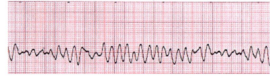

   a. Ventricular fibrillation
   b. Atrial fibrillation
   c. Atrial flutter
   d. Normal sinus rhythm

50. When the PR interval is prolonged and greater than .02 seconds it is called:
   a. Second degree heart block type I
   b. First degree heart block type I
   c. Third degree heart block type I
   d. Fourth degree heart block type I

51. A complete heart block occurs when:
   a. Impulses generated by the SA node do not reach the ventricular fibers
   b. Impulses generated by the AV node do not reach the atrial fibers
   c. The heart does not completely depolarize
   d. The heart does not completely repolarize

52. The following is an example of

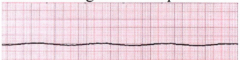

   a. Supraventricular tachycardia
   b. Atrial fibrillation
   c. Sinus fibrillation
   d. Asystole

53. Which of the following are characterized by saw toothed waves?
   a. Atrial flutter
   b. Asystole
   c. Sinus flutter

d. Ventricular tachycardia

54. During stress and exercise which of the following is normal?
    a. Bradycardia
    b. Tachycardia
    c. Asystole
    d. Flutter

55. The following is an example of

    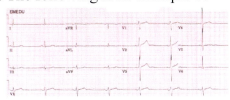

    a. A normal sinus rhythm
    b. Sinus bradycardia
    c. Sinus tachycardia
    d. Sinus flutter

56. The baseline method of analyzing the EKG involves:
    a. Comparing P waves and QRS complexes first
    b. Identifying normal behavior of the heart for comparison
    c. Comparing EKGs to older EKGs
    d. None of the above

57. The normal duration for the QRS complex is:
    a. Less than .2 seconds
    b. Less than .18 seconds
    c. Less than .12 seconds
    d. Less than .08 seconds

58. The vertical axis of the EKG represents:
    a. Time
    b. Blood flow
    c. Voltage
    d. Blood pressure

59. What does not appear on an EKG?
    a. Ventricular repolarization
    b. AV repolarization
    c. SA repolarization
    d. Atrial repolarization

60. Which of the following is true about the T wave?
    a. Represents repolarization of Purkinje fibers
    b. It represents the time of ventricular contraction
    c. It is slightly asymmetric
    d. It represent ventricular activity

61. Complex or diverse could possible represent:
    a. Impulses could be passing along wrong pathways
    b. Impulses are travelling the proper path
    c. Impulses are strong and normal
    d. All of the above

62. Where is the J junction?
    a. Where the QRS complex ends and the ST segment begins
    b. Where the ST complex ends and the UV wave begins
    c. Where the PQR complex ends and the ST segment begins

d. None of the above

63. The following is an example of

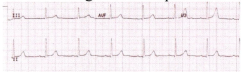

   a. Sinus bradycardia
   b. Sinus tachycardia
   c. Normal sinus rhythm
   d. Sinus arrhythmia

64. What is the first deflection after diastole?
   a. The QRS wave
   b. The T wave
   c. The P wave
   d. The Q wave

65. Which node regulates heartrate?
   a. AV node
   b. Purkinje fibers
   c. SM node
   d. SA node

66. Five small squares on the EKG represents:
   a. .1 seconds
   b. .2 seconds
   c. .3 seconds
   d. .4 seconds

67. Five large squares on the EKG represents:
   a. 1 second
   b. 2 seconds
   c. 3 seconds
   d. 4 seconds

68. Resting cells are:
   a. Neutrally charged
   b. Negatively charged
   c. Positively charged
   d. None of the above

69. A complete heart block occurs when:
   a. Impulses generated by the SA node do not reach the ventricular fibers
   b. Impulses generated by the AV node do not reach the atrial fibers
   c. The heart does not completely depolarize
   d. The heart does not completely repolarize

70. Diseases of valves are called:
   a. Hums
   b. Murmurs
   c. Skips
   d. Beats

71. Conductivity refers to:
   a. Irritability of cells
   b. The ability of cells to shorten and expand
   c. The ability of cells to receive and send electrical stimulus
   d. The ability of the heart to regulate itself

72. The first heart sound is the result of:
   a. The aortic and pulmonic valves closing
   b. The mitral and tricuspid valves closing

c. The capillaries closing
d. The heart contracting

73. The second heart sound is the result of:
a. The aortic and pulmonic valves closing
b. The mitral and tricuspid valves closing
c. The capillaries closing
d. The heart contracting

74. How many chambers to the heart have?
a. 3 chambers
b. 5 chambers
c. 2 chambers
d. 4 chambers

75. During a stress test the patient exercises by:
a. Doing jumping jacks
b. Doing sit ups
c. Chair aerobics
d. Running on a treadmill

76. Which test monitor's the patient's heart readings for an entire day?
a. Stress test
b. Holter monitor
c. EKG
d. Cardiological movement test

77. Who analyzes the heart rhythms recorded on an EKG?
a. Medical Assistant
b. Cardiologist
c. EKG Technician
d. Registered Nurse

78. Who positions the patient and prepares him/her for the test?
a. Medical Assistant
b. Cardiologist
c. EKG Technician
d. Registered Nurse

79. Which kind of tissue forms the largest part of the heart?
a. Myocardial tissue
b. Endocardial tissue
c. Endothelial tissue
d. A combination of all of the above

80. The inner part of the heart is referred to as:
a. Myocardium
b. Endocardium
c. Epicardium
d. Endotheilium

81. How long does a patient wear a Holter monitor?
a. A day
b. A week
c. 6 hours
d. 3 hours

82. When an electrical impulse originates from somewhere other than the SA node it is called:
a. A normal sinus rhythm
b. Ectopic rhythm
c. Conduction block
d. Pre-excitation syndrome

83. Which part of the heart receives oxygenated blood?

a. Right atrium
b. Right ventricle
c. Left atrium
d. Left ventricle

84. Which of the following statements is true?
a. The atria contract together
b. The ventricles contract together
c. The atria do not contract at the same time as the ventricles
d. All of the above

85. Which of the following are also known as semi-lunar valves?
a. Pulmonic valves
b. Mitral valves
c. Tricuspid valves
d. Aortic valves

86. Contracting _____ create systolic pressure.
a. Ventricles
b. Atria
c. Capillaries
d. Veins

87. Which of the following causes diastole?
a. Contracting atria
b. Contracting ventricles
c. Relaxing atria
d. Relaxing ventricles

88. Which of the following receives impulses directly from the SA node?
a. Purkinje fibers
b. Jugular node
c. AV node
d. Bundle of HIS

89. The QT interval:
a. Shows all atrial activity
b. Represents all ventricular activity
c. Shows all Sinoatrial activity
d. Represents all Cardiac activity

90. Which segment is compared to the PR segment to identify ischemia or injury?
a. ST segment
b. QT segment
c. QRS complex
d. RST complex

91. Which test is performed while the patient is on a treadmill in order to provide readings at diversified physical force?
a. The CT test
b. The Physical
c. The Stress test
d. The Psychological test

92. Which of the following sets the pace for the heartbeat?
a. The AV node
b. The ventricular node
c. The atrial node
d. The SA node

93. When an impulse encounters blocks or delays it is called:

a. Pre-excitation syndrome
b. Conduction block
c. Normal SA node
d. Tachycardia

94. Which veins carry oxygenated blood?
    a. Jugular veins
    b. Pulmonary veins
    c. Coronary veins
    d. Vessical veins

95. When an impulse originates from the AV node it is called:
    a. An ectopic rhythm
    b. A conduction block
    c. Pulmonary block
    d. A Sinus rhythm

96. What is it called when complexes are greater than 0.12 sec with a slurred up strike (delta wave) seen in one or more leads?
    a. SA reentry tachycardia
    b. AV reentry tachycardia
    c. SA reentry bradycardia
    d. AV reentry bradycardia

97. Which of the following can cause sinus tachycardia?
    a. Caffeine
    b. Fever
    c. Exercise
    d. All of the above

98. Which of the following can be said about sinus bradycardia?
    a. It normally occurs during sleep
    b. It can be normal for athletes
    c. It is decreased bloodflow to the body
    d. All of the above

99. A stimulated cell is:
    a. Positively charged
    b. Negatively charged
    c. Neutrally charged
    d. None of the above

100. When multiple electrical impulses occur across the heart it causes:
    a. Sinus rhythm
    b. Asytole
    c. Ventricular rhythm
    d. Quiver

Answers for Section Two

1. B
2. D
3. C
4. B
5. C
6. B
7. D

8.	D		45.	B
9.	B		46.	A
10.	C		47.	C
11.	B		48.	D
12.	A		49.	A
13.	B		50.	B
14.	C		51.	A
15.	D		52.	D
16.	C		53.	A
17.	C		54.	B
18.	D		55.	B
19.	C		56.	B
20.	B		57.	C
21.	A		58.	C
22.	B		59.	D
23.	C		60.	C
24.	B		61.	A
25.	A		62.	A
26.	D		63.	C
27.	B		64.	C
28.	D		65.	D
29.	A		66.	B
30.	C		67.	A
31.	B		68.	B
32.	A		69.	A
33.	D		70.	B
34.	D		71.	C
35.	B		72.	B
36.	A		73.	A
37.	B		74.	D
38.	A		75.	D
39.	C		76.	B
40.	B		77.	B
41.	C		78.	C
42.	D		79.	A
43.	C		80.	B
44.	B		81.	A

82. B
83. C
84. D
85. B
86. A
87. D
88. C
89. B
90. A
91. C
92. D
93. B
94. B
95. A
96. B
97. D
98. D
99. A
100. D

**Good Luck in Your Exams!
Go in with confidence…And Pass!!**

Made in the USA
Columbia, SC
23 October 2022